30 CHINESE DINNERS
HEALTHY EASY HOMEMADE MEALS

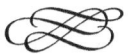

I. NGEOW

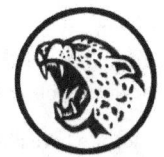

ISBN 978-1-913584-04-7

Copyright © 2020 by I. Ngeow

All rights reserved.

No part of this book may be reproduced in any form or by any electronic or mechanical means, including information storage and retrieval systems, without written permission from the author, except for the use of brief quotations in a book review.

Written and illustrated by I. Ngeow, except where photo credit is given.

For my mother and my late grandmothers

CONTENTS

Foreword — vii
Introduction — ix
Before we begin — xiii

1. Special Fried Rice — 1
2. Egg fried rice — 4
3. Char Siew Roast Pork — 6
4. Chicken, red pepper and broccoli in oyster sauce — 10
5. Grilled salmon, vegetables and soba noodles — 13
6. Steamed egg and mince (Hakka egg) — 16
7. Lemon Chicken — 18
8. Monk's Vegetables (Buddha's Delight) — 21
9. My mum's eggplant (brinjal) with shrimp — 23
10. Shrimp or Prawn bee hoon (rice vermicelli) — 26
11. Vegan Bee Hoon — 28
12. My mum's Kung Pao Chi Ting (Kung Po Chicken) — 30
13. Vegan Chow Mein — 34
14. Woh Tip (Pot Stickers/ Pan Stickers) — 36
15. Just plain regular light and crispy tofu — 40
16. My mum's Marmite Chicken — 42
17. Hong Kong Chinese Chives Omelette — 45
18. Shrimp and Chinese cabbage tagliatelle — 47
19. Singapore Prawn Noodle Soup (Hei Mee) — 49
20. Hakka claypot mince pork and tofu — 52
21. Chicken Chow Mein — 55
22. Three mushroom tofu — 58
23. Aubergine (eggplant) Thai red curry and cauliflower rice — 61
24. My daughter's 5-ingredient Chicken in 10 minutes — 64
25. My granny's minced pork with noodles (Hakka mein) — 67
26. Chicken macaroni soup (slow cooker) — 69
27. Sweet and Sour Meatballs (or Fish) — 71
28. Steamed Seabass in 15 minutes — 76

29. Crispy Roast duck with pancakes	78
30. Blanched pak choy	82
31. Beef hor fun (flat rice noodles)	84
32. 5-ingredient shrimp and green beans in 10 minutes	87
33. Red bean soup (dessert)	89
34. How to make perfect rice	91
35. Top 3 essential DIY marinades, sauces & pastes	93
36. List of recipes	95
Before you go	97
About the Author	99
Also by I. Ngeow	101
Acknowledgments	103

FOREWORD

Ivy Ngeow is a multi-talented architect whose skill stretches beyond designs of buildings. With creativity hard-wired in her DNA, she is an accomplished author of three novels and short stories, a musician, fashionista, artist, keep-fit guru and cook. A devoted mother to her two children, she creates many dishes to cater for her family.

If you are trying to find recipes to cook at home, help is at hand with Ivy's handy cookbook *30 Chinese Dinners* with easy homemade family meal recipes readily available from supermarkets along with explanation of each dish.

Ivy Ngeow hails from Malaysia where food is a national preoccupation. With a population of largely immigrants from the four corners of the world, Malaysian food and drinks can aptly be described as an Asian melting-pot. Each migratory population from China, India, Middle East and Europe along with the indigenous populace contribute to the gastronomic culture of Malaysia today. Against this background, Ivy imparts her local knowledge on the art of cooking Malaysian Chinese dishes she learned from her grandmothers growing up in Malaysia.

FOREWORD

So, let the culinary adventure begin with Ivy Ngeow's cookbook *30 Chinese Dinners* and get cooking.

Helen Oon

———

ABOUT HELEN OON

Helen Oon is a Malaysian-born travel writer and amateur cook based in the United Kingdom. With over thirty years of experience in the travel industry, she became a professional travel writer in 1994 writing freelance for magazines, newspapers and online travel websites. She has written six travel guides to Malaysia, Singapore and Hong Kong for New Holland Publishers Ltd (UK). Her travel blog, My Faces and Places (https://myfacesandplaces.co.uk) features her travel journeys around the world. One of her passions is cooking which she finds therapeutic and social-enhancing.

INTRODUCTION

- AND A BIT ABOUT ME -

I WROTE THIS BOOK because I don't like cooking. I know! Right? You cannot believe you are reading this. It's true. I like made up, adapted easy meals. This book is intended for both Chinese and non-Chinese cooks at all levels of cooking skills. The objective is that everyone can have a go at making a homemade Chinese meal. It avoids wasting food, money and time. It's actually quicker to throw a meal together than to order a takeout or a takeaway.

The idea for this book came about after my Instagram photos of healthy dinners and meals I make for my family became highly popular. Friends and followers have asked me for recipes. I don't use any recipes as I know these meals by heart and they are made from the heart. All I know is that they are tasty and perfect for the time-poor. If they work for me they will work for you.

I don't do 'this' cooking or 'that' cooking. I have no particular formal method and I am not a trained chef or cook. I am a mother, author, architect, makeup artist and musician. All these creative journeys have given me the experience and the maturity to trust my creative instincts and my no-nonsense approach to the kitchen.

INTRODUCTION

This book is non halal and non kosher. Feel free to substitute the pork with turkey, meat with quorn, textured vegetable protein (TVP) or vegetarian products. My system is flexible.

Most of these meals are standard traditional homemade Malaysian Chinese meals which my grandmothers and my mum made with thrift and Asian frugality to feed the family. My paternal grandmother was Hakka, which was the only nomadic tribe in China and never bound women's feet. Because of the tradition of travelling, walking and making temporary homes, Hakka food is usually meaty, rich with preserved vegetables, or totally vegetarian because there might be only one or the other at any point in time.

My maternal grandmother was Hokkien. The Chinese in Singapore and Malaysia are mostly from south China as they arrived during the Great Famine in China in the 1920s to work as labourers in Singapore and Malaysia. Hokkiens make up a large part of the original Chinese immigrant population. In fact the word for labourer in Hokkien is *ku li* which is derivative of the English word *coolie*, which in turn originated from the Hindi *kuli* (labourer) or Urdu *kuli* (slave). As a third generation Chinese born and raised in Johor Bahru, I had a basic childhood as my city was huge, industrial and grim. It still is, but it's now commercialised too. I digress.

My entire family background, and that of all Chinese immigrants to Singapore and Malaysia from the interwar period, is working class. My city of Johor Bahru is almost all working class even today. Ask anyone local to my city and they will tell you it's all nail salons, car washes, restaurants, bridal shops, factories, pineapple plantations, rubber estates, mega malls, supermarkets and office blocks. There are 9 colleges and universities.

We provide the work force for Singapore due to the vast currency difference. As a result of generations of poverty and hardship, nothing was thrown away. Every leftover or morsel could be modified into another meal or two. Every huge or oversized serving could be halved and turned into another meal again. Every upcycling was a creative or re-inventive process. These meals were made without any precise measurements, a process called *agak-agak*, which is Malay for guesstimating. Hence in the ingredients list you will find terms like a splash of wine, an inch of ginger, a squirt of honey. I have adapted the use of the traditional meals for modern purposes and of course for ease of acquiring the Asian ingredients in a Western-style supermarket, society and community. In the past, meals were made fresh rather than frozen in bulk for future use. Of course that had to change with modern lifestyles. No one has the time to shop every day in a wet market for fresh food.

The terminology in this book is both in US and UK English. I guess that covers you guys or most of you in the world.

When you follow the recipes, feel free to adjust or ignore the suggested amount size in the ingredient list. You can do all of it by taste and according to your dietary requirement. For example, I increase the protein and the vegetable content and decrease the fat, carb and the salt in every meal. This is to promote healthy living and eating. If you like to go low fat, low salt and high protein too, then great! Just go with my recommended amounts.

My top tip for you in Chinese cooking lies in preparation. It is 95% preparation and 5% cooking. By this I mean firstly in the size of the pieces you are cutting, chopping, dicing, slicing etc and secondly, the marinades. There is no oven to even out the appearance of the meal or to delay the cooking process. The complete meal is not cooked whole unlike in Western cooking. The sum of the equation is more important than the finished product. Marinating and cutting ingredients to the correct size is mandatory in Chinese cooking. This is to do with the short cooking time. Too large and it will not cook properly. Too small and it will burn or be overcooked. Not marinating will lead to hard and tasteless chunks of food. You will not be able to achieve that glossy or velvety delicate flavour symbolic of Chinese food. How do you know what the correct size is? Look at the photos. The proportion of each item to another will tell you.

INTRODUCTION

I have included one dessert (red bean soup) and a couple of side dishes (pak choy and egg fried rice) to make 33 recipes in total.

One last thing. If what you cook from this book doesn't taste like something from a restaurant or a takeaway, then congratulations, you did it. It means you have made real homemade and healthy Chinese food. With less salt and grease, and zero MSG, it should taste superior to a restaurant or takeaway meal.

Have fun and let's start!

BEFORE WE BEGIN

THIS IS A LIST of the basic tools, store cupboard and fridge ingredients you will need before you start any simple Chinese meal. Without these you are asking for trouble. You will waste time and the meals will taste wrong. Do you really want to boil and strain rice and burn the bottom of the pot? Rice is not pasta. A plasterer cannot plaster the wall using a butter knife. Therefore, always use the right equipment and ingredient list.

Do not be daunted by the list. In the equipment list, you only ever need one spatula, one knife and one pan (the wok). You will very rarely need wooden spoons, ladle, scoops, pans or pots. One wok, one spatula and one knife do all the tasks required in Chinese cooking.

ELECTRICAL APPLIANCES

- Rice cooker
- Hand blender or mini chopper (optional)
- Air fryer (optional)

EQUIPMENT

- Spatula
- Wok
- Chopper knife (cleaver)
- Steaming rack (optional)

STORE CUPBOARD INGREDIENTS

- Fish sauce
- Soy sauce
- Dark soy sauce
- Hoisin sauce
- Plum sauce
- White pepper
- Dried shrimps, ha mai or xia mi, minced into breadcrumb consistency (optional)
- Dry fried onions
- Crumbed dried salted fish, ham yu, kiam hu or xian yu, (optional)
- Five spice powder
- Sesame oil
- Chinese cooking wine — I use Shaoxing wine and you may substitute with sherry
- Rice wine vinegar — I substitute with white wine vinegar
- Ketchup
- Oyster sauce
- Chilli powder
- Dried chilli flakes
- Sweet chilli sauce eg Blue Dragon or Thai sweet chilli
- Garlic chilli sauce eg Sriracha
- Breadcrumbs (Panko or ordinary)
- Cornflour
- Plain flour or wheat flour

- Tapioca flour or rice flour

FRIDGE INGREDIENTS

- Ginger and garlic in a jar (minced, ready as a paste)
- Garlic in a jar (minced, ready as a paste)
- Dry fried garlic crumbs (to make your own: toast or air fry cloves of garlic and bash them down into a breadcrumb consistency)

SPECIAL FRIED RICE

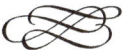

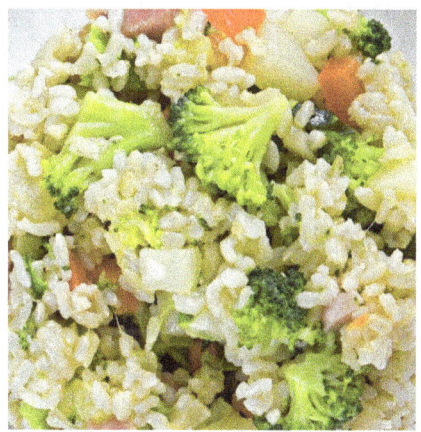

This was the first meal I made as a 12-year-old. It is an "every" meal. In Asia, it could be eaten for breakfast, lunch, snack or dinner. It is another classic frugal family dish because it involves upcycling any small amount of leftovers which at first may not seem enough to feed everyone. But once thrown together, the "sum of the parts is more than the whole". I am able to rustle this up when my children come home starving from school as a snack, or in the morning for my daughter's packed lunch while I'm drinking coffee at breakfast. It takes only 10 minutes. Remember the golden rule:

"If it's taking too long, something is wrong."

- Ivy Ngeow

Serves 2-4

- 2 tbsp oil for frying like rice bran oil (or another healthy alternative)
- 1 egg
- 2 stalks of scallions (spring onions), chopped finely. Separate the white and the green parts.
- 1 to 1½ cup of vegetables eg frozen mixed vegetables with cauliflower, peas and carrots, diced mushrooms and/or peppers. Anything colourful. If you have nothing, peas will do.
- ½ to 1 cup of chopped protein eg char siew, ham, chorizo, hotdog, chicken, firm tofu or shrimp/prawn
- 2 cups cold brown, white or mixed rice (cooked rice from the day before). See chapter on How to Make Perfect Rice first.
- Dry fried onions and the green part of spring onions to garnish.
- A splash of fish sauce or soy sauce, and pepper to taste

1. Heat the oil until hot. Sauté the white parts of the scallions (spring onions) until fragrant which is about 2-3 minutes.
2. Add vegetables and sauté for 2-3 minutes, if they are cooked already. If they are raw, sauté for another 2 minutes. Do not add water. Other recipes ask you to do that because the vegetables have not been chopped up enough and as a result are unable to cook quickly.
3. Add the meat and sauté for 1 minute.
4. Add rice and sauté for 1 minute. Make a well in the centre and add the egg, beating it all the time like making scrambled eggs

in the centre of the well. When it is cooked and not liquid anymore, then only fold the rice in all directions towards the centre.
5. Garnish with the dry fried onions and a few slices of the green part of the scallions/spring onions sprinkled over the rice when serving.
6. Splash on fish sauce or soy sauce, and pepper to taste.

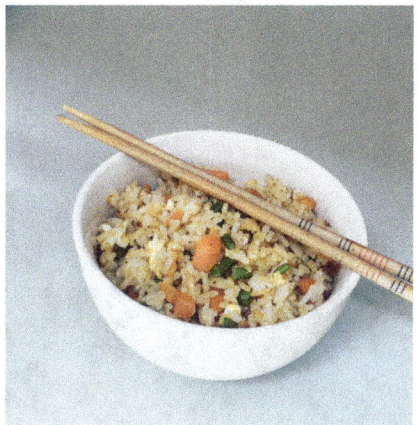

EGG FRIED RICE

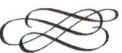

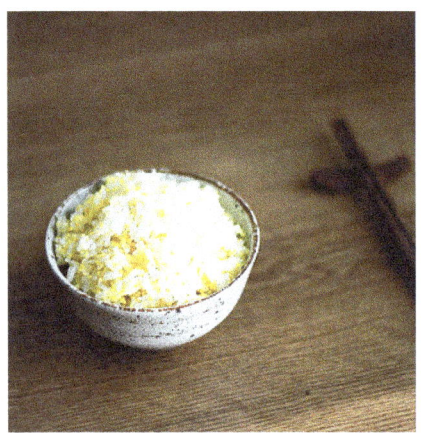

An EVEN easier variation and a vegetarian option. My son actually prefers this to special fried rice. This is a great recipe that is so tasty when there is nothing else to eat in the house, for example, when I was a student, or for beginners to cooking, like children. It will take you about 5 minutes.

Serves 2-4

- 2 tbsp oil for frying like rice bran oil (or another healthy alternative)
- 2 eggs
- 1 cup of vegetables eg frozen peas
- 2 cups cold brown, white or mixed rice (cooked rice from the day before)
- Dry fried onions OR a pinch of crumbed salted fish to garnish
- A splash of soy sauce, and pepper to taste
- Optional: red chillies thinly sliced

1. Heat the oil until hot. Add rice and sauté for 1 minute.
2. Add frozen peas and sauté for 2-3 minutes. Add the eggs, beating them all the time like making scrambled eggs in the centre of the well. When it is cooked and not liquid anymore, then only fold the rice in all directions towards the centre.
3. Garnish with the dry fried onions or the crumbed salted fish and the optional sliced red chillies. Splash on soy sauce and pepper to taste. Put in bowl. Eat on your lap at the TV. Bliss.

CHAR SIEW ROAST PORK

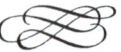

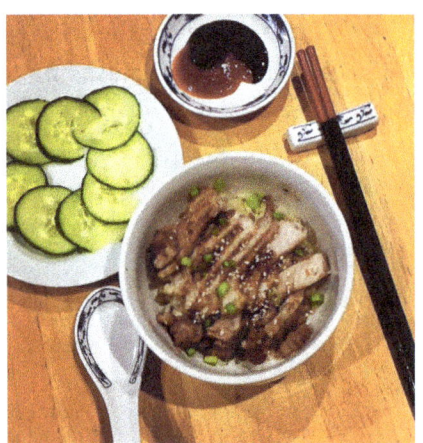

This is a very versatile roast dish. It can be added to other meals such as Special Fried Rice. It can be served plain with boiled rice and a cucumber salad (my favourite meal when I was a schoolgirl). It can be made in advance and frozen. It can also be a filling for buns (Char Siew Pau), dumplings and pastries. You can also buy "Chinese tacos" which is the moon-shaped white *bao* and from there make a sandwich type snack. I have used it as a salad topping too for low carb meals.

Serves 6

- 2 tsp ginger and garlic paste
- 1 splash of Shaoxing wine
- 1 tbsp oyster sauce
- 1 dsp five spice powder
- 1 splash sesame oil
- 1 tsp chilli powder
- 1 splash soy sauce
- Squirt of honey
- Dash of white pepper
- 1 lbs or 450g of pork chop, fillet, or loin steaks
- Thinly sliced scallions/spring onions and minced coriander for garnish.
- Squirt of hoisin sauce in squeezy bottle

1. Put all of the above except the last two in a covered big bowl or plastic bag. Leave for 4 hours or overnight in fridge.
2. Preheat open to 190 deg C (375 deg F or gas mark 5).
3. Turn the grill to full and grill for 5 minutes to brown the meat and seal it. Turn the meat half way. Switch off the grill.
4. Place meat on a wire rack of a roasting dish. Roast for 20 minutes, checking during the half way mark and turning if required.
5. Remove the pork. Put on a large cutting board and allow to cool for 5-10 minutes before slicing thinly. Arrange on a big flat plate in rows in an orderly manner using the blade of the knife to move the rows. Don't dump the whole lot of char siew in a disorganised pile.
6. Squirt the hoisin from the squeeze bottle in a drizzly zigzag (or whatever artistic style you feel the urge to create) over the beautifully-arranged sliced char siew. Top that with a flourish of the scallions/spring onions and minced coriander garnish. Serve hot or cold as per suggestions given.

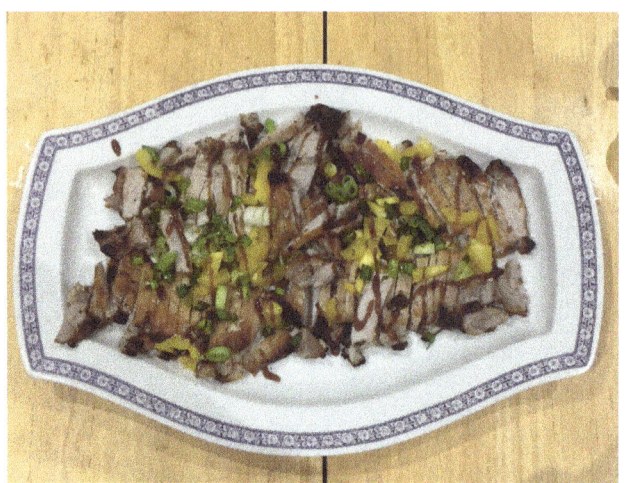

Serve on large dish as a special occasion main meal to share

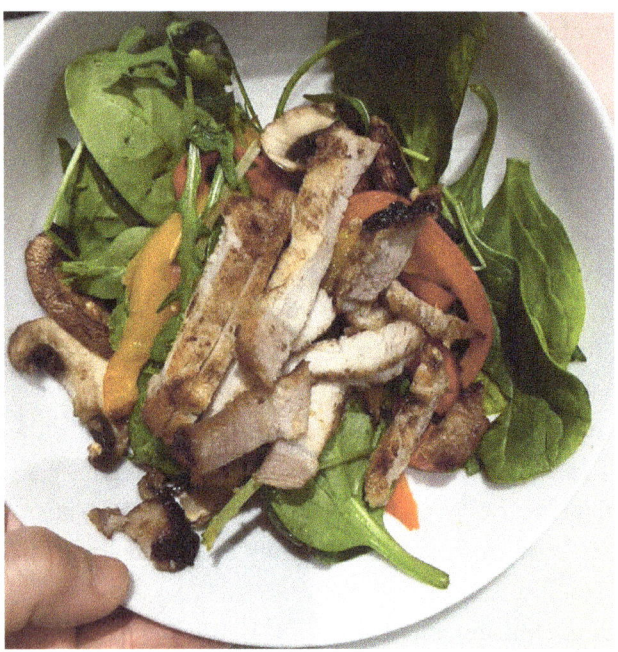

Serve on green leafy salad as low carb, high protein, high fibre meal.

30 CHINESE DINNERS

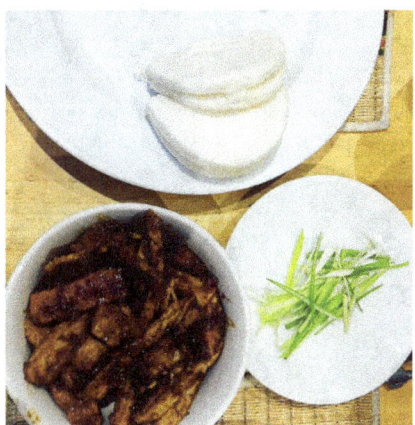

Eat with "bao" like Chinese tacos

CHICKEN, RED PEPPER AND BROCCOLI IN OYSTER SAUCE

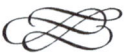

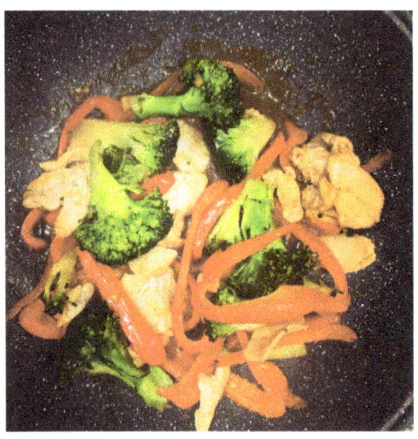

This meal can be made in 12 minutes. I know because I have had exactly this amount of time to prepare it before my daughter's ballet.

HOT TIP #1: substitute the chicken with thinly-sliced beef. **HOT TIP #2:** the first 4 ingredients below are the Fab Four[1]. It is the basic building block of Chinese cooking. The oyster sauce can also be soy sauce if you are vegan, or you don't eat any seafood products.

HOT TIP #3: Garnish with or add thinly-sliced red chillies.

Serves 2-4

- 2 tsp ginger and garlic paste
- 1 splash of Shaoxing wine
- 1 dsp oyster sauce
- 1 splash sesame oil
- 1 dsp cornflour
- 2 chicken breasts thinly sliced
- 1 red pepper
- 1 small to medium broccoli
- 1 tsp dark soy sauce
- 2 tbsp oil for frying like rice bran oil (or another healthy alternative)

For the sauce:

- ½ cup of water
- 1 tsp bicarbonate of soda
- 1 tsp of cornflour
- 1 tsp dark soy sauce

1. Dump the first 6 ingredients into a big bowl and mix well. Leave this, covered. **HOT TIP #4:** If you can, leave it marinaded for a few hours in the fridge to create a velvety texture and professional finesse to the chicken. But if you are a busy mum like me, and you forgot to prep earlier, then never mind. Just leave it for 2 minutes while you get on with the rest of the steps.
2. Slice the red pepper thinly. Pluck the broccoli florets by hand, no chopping required. Cut crosses in the stalks which are thick, so that they will cook quicker. Peel and thinly slice into rectangles or ovals the rest of the abandoned stalk (the "tree trunk" of the broccoli that's left). Chinese people never waste

the trunk. It's all fibre.
3. Mix half a cup of water, a tsp of bicarbonate of soda, a teaspoon of cornflour and a teaspoon of dark soy sauce. Leave.
4. Heat 2 tbsp of oil in a wok until hot. Pour in the mixture from the big bowl. Sauté for 2 minutes until chicken is browned.
5. Add all the vegetables and sauté for 2 minutes. Add a splash of water. Cover with the wok lid and steam for 3 minutes. Open the lid and add the cornflour and water mixture. Stir again for a minute or until the sauce thickens. Do not replace the lid. Serve out immediately to keep freshness and the colour.
6. Serve with wholewheat noodles or rice. Or if you are going low carb, serve with a pile of green salad such as spinach and tomatoes with a handful of mixed unsalted nuts.

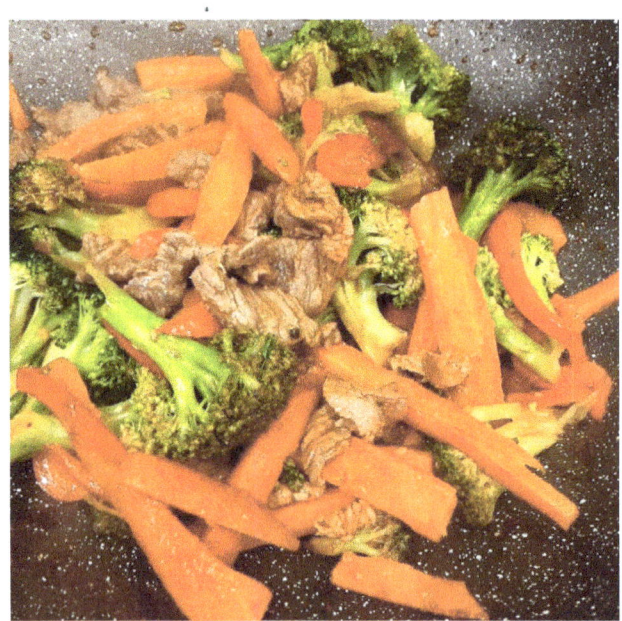

Hot tip: substitute with beef

---

1. See the section at the end on *Top 3 essential DIY marinades, sauces and pastes*.

GRILLED SALMON, VEGETABLES AND SOBA NOODLES

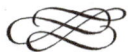

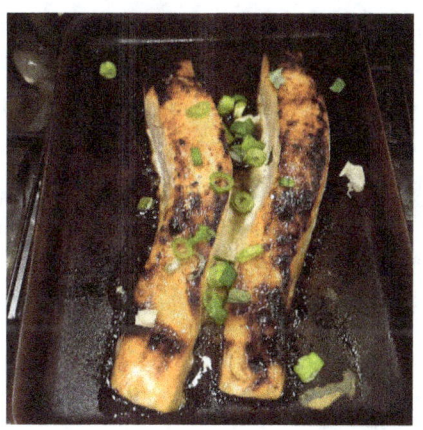

This is a healthy meal full of Omega 3. You can actually eat this for breakfast too and it will really set you up, mind and body, for the whole day.

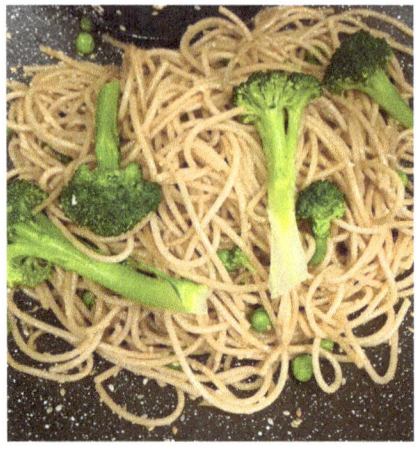

HOT TIP #1: You can substitute the soba or buckwheat noodles with wholewheat spaghetti. No one will know! Still very easy, tasty and *al dente*. **HOT TIP #2:** Prepare in advance the sesame seeds and keep in an airtight jar. You can use them as a topping in a variety of meals as a topping or garnish. Toast them in an oven or lightly dry fry in a small frying pan without oil for a few seconds. Watch that they don't burn. **HOT TIP #3:** Prepare the marinade[1] in advance and store in the fridge in a jar. You can save time by using this over and over in different meals without having to prepare each time. I do it each time because I don't have enough space in the fridge and it does not take long as I do not measure any of the ingredients anymore. I do it by eye.

Serves 4

The Fab Four marinade

- 1 tsp minced garlic and ginger paste from the jar
- A splash of sesame oil
- A splash of Shaoxing wine
- A few drops of oyster or soy sauce

The other ingredients

- 4 pieces of fresh Atlantic salmon marinaded in the Fab Four (see above) in the fridge for at least 4 hours or overnight.
- A squirt of honey from a squeezy bottle
- A few drops of dark soy sauce
- Sliced scallions/spring onions, the green part, for garnish
- Toasted sesame seeds
- 2-3 packets of soba noodles or buckwheat noodles.
- 1 broccoli, florets plucked off from the main tree trunk by hand.

1. Preheat grill to maximum.
2. Cook the noodles according to the instructions. Drain and set aside.
3. Heat water in a saucepan until boiling. Add the broccoli florets and boil for 4 minutes. Remove from heat and drain immediately to prevent overcooking. The green should be bright and lurid, and the stems soft when you stab a sharp knife into them.
4. Put the salmon on a grilling metal tray or dish and sparingly drizzle over dark soy sauce and honey (in that order). Grill for 3-5 minutes or until slightly browned and crispy. Switch off grill and leave the salmon there.
5. Toss the broccoli, sesame seeds and the noodles in a large mixing bowl with a splash of sesame oil. Using tongs or large chopsticks, grab the mixture and serve into bowls.
6. Place salmon on top of each bowl and garnish with the spring onions.

---

1. See the section at the end on *Top 3 essential DIY marinades, sauces and pastes.*

STEAMED EGG AND MINCE (HAKKA EGG)

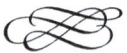

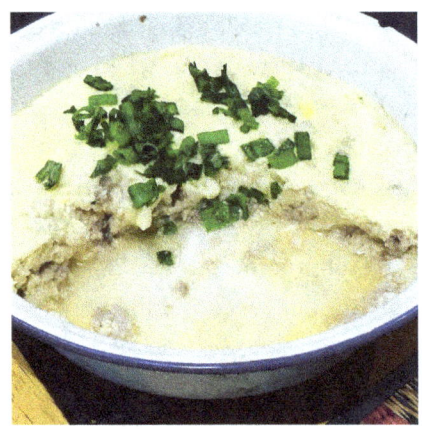

I grew up eating this meal as it was one the classics that my paternal grandmother (Por Por) made. Therefore it has fond memories of early childhood for me. I remember being able to smell the egg steaming as I came home from school.

Serves 3-4

- 8" diameter and 2" deep metal enamel or stainless steel dish and steaming rack
- 3 eggs
- ½ cup of minced pork
- Marinade (see Fab Four in top 3 essential DIY marinades, sauces and pastes) for at least four hours if possible, if not a few minutes
- White pepper
- ½ a cup of milk or dairy-free alternative
- Chopped coriander and crumbed salted fish for garnish

1. Beat the eggs and place in the steaming dish. Add mince and using a fork flatten the mince roughly and loosely. Add a dash of pepper.
2. Place dish on steaming rack in the wok. Fill the wok with water to a third. Steam for at least 15 minutes. Test by poking a knife in to the dish to check that the meat is fully cooked.
3. Garnish with coriander and crumbed salted fish. Serve with rice or vegetables if on low carb.

LEMON CHICKEN

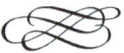

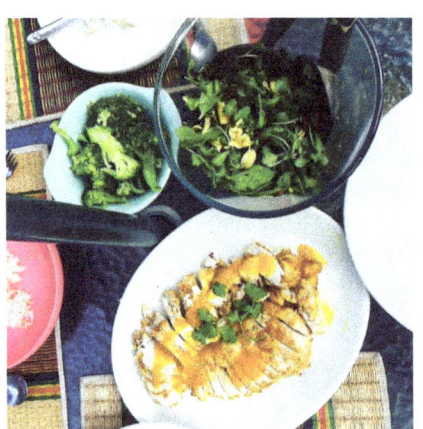

This is another family classic that my children love. **HOT TIP #1:** Traditionally rich and deep fried, my low-fat version here uses skinless chicken and air frying. The egg and cornflour batter will taste light and crispy. If you do not have an air fryer, you can oven cook at the same temperature and time as below. **HOT TIP #2**: slice the chicken breast horizontally to turn each breast into two. Save money, eat less, double the chicken. Win-win.

Serves 4

- 2 skinless chicken breasts, patted dry with paper towel if wet
- 1 egg (beaten)
- 2 tbsp cornflour
- 1 tbsp rice bran oil or another healthy alternative

For the lemon sauce

- 2 tbsp lemon juice
- 1 tsp ground turmeric
- 1 tbsp sugar or ½ tsp Stevia
- 1 tbsp plum sauce
- 1 dsp cornflour
- 3 quarter cup water
- Coriander leaves on stalk for garnish

1. Preheat air fryer or oven if you have no air fryer to 190 deg C or 375 deg F.
2. Slice chicken horizontally or latitudinally. Dip the 4 escalopes in the egg and then the cornflour. Put it back into the egg and then the cornflour again.
3. In a frying pan, fry the escalopes lightly for about 2 minutes to brown both sides. Remove and place in air fryer or oven for 18 minutes. While it is in the air fryer or oven, make the sauce.
4. Add all the sauce ingredients to a saucepan. Bring to a simmer. Keep stirring until the sauce thickens. Switch off the heat.
5. Take chicken out of oven or air fryer and place on wooden chopping board. Allow to cool for about 2 minutes before cutting into 1" strips. Place neatly in rows on a serving dish and not in a disorderly pile. Aim to still be able to tell the original shape of the escalope.
6. Drizzle or pour the sauce over and serve with fresh coriander leaves. Eat with rice and vegetables or if on low carb, eat with

edamame and quinoa green salad. **HOT TIP #3**: The sauce can also be a salad dressing. If you have leftovers, you can keep it for another day or use.

MONK'S VEGETABLES (BUDDHA'S DELIGHT)

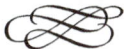

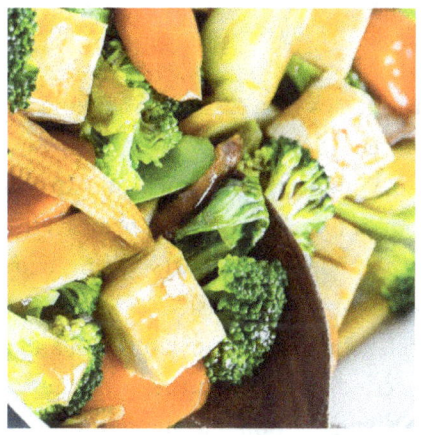

This dish is called Monk's Vegetables or Buddha's Delight because Chinese monks are vegetarians. Lotus root, fresh or tinned, is available in Chinese supermarkets. **HOT TIP:** If you can get some, try replacing the firm tofu with dried tofu (fu chok) strips, soaked in hot water for an hour. It's much tastier and full of texture due to the stringy fibrous texture.

Serves 4

1. NGEOW

- ½ cup of firm tofu, cut into batons
- One third cup of wood ear (dried cloud ears) fungus soaked in hot water for 15 minutes
- 8 dried Chinese or shiitake mushrooms soaked in hot water for 15 minutes
- 1 tbsp rice bran oil or another healthy alternative
- ½ cup lotus root, peeled and sliced
- ¾ cup tinned straw mushrooms, washed and drained
- 1 cup baby corn, sliced in half longitudinally
- One third cup of mange tout or snow peas
- A splash of light soy sauce
- A splash of Shaoxing wine
- ½ tsp of Stevia or 2 tsp of sugar
- 1 tsp of vegetable stock powder mixed with two-third cup warm water
- 1 tsp cornflour

1. Mix the cornflour, soy sauce, sugar, Shaoxing wine and stock in a jug and leave aside.
2. Drain both the wood ear and Chinese mushrooms. Cut off the hard and woody stalks. Slice the mushrooms thinly.
3. Heat oil in a wok add the wood ears, Chinese mushrooms and lotus road. Sauté for 30 seconds.
4. Add the tofu, straw mushrooms, baby corn and mange tout. Sauté for 3o seconds. Add a third cup of water and replace the lid on the wok. Bring to boil and steam the contents for 3 minutes.
5. Open the lid and add the sauce mixture, stirring until it thickens. Serve hot.

MY MUM'S EGGPLANT (BRINJAL) WITH SHRIMP

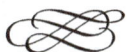

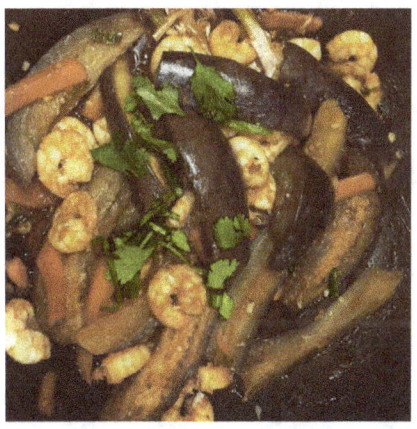

This is a classic meal whenever I go home to Johor Bahru. I can eat this three times a day and every day. Aubergine/eggplant/brinjal is definitely one of my favourite vegetables. **HOT TIP:** use the Asian brinjal from Chinese supermarkets if you can. If you cannot find this, you may substitute with the Western aubergine/eggplant.

Serves 2-4

- 2 cloves of garlic, chopped
- 1 aubergine/eggplant/brinjal
- ½ cup of little shrimp cooked or raw
- A few drops of oyster sauce
- ½ cup of chopped coriander
- Sliced red chillies
- Rice bran oil for frying

- Cut the aubergine/eggplant/brinjal into half at first (transverse, latitudinal or cross section). Then, the bottom is to be cut into 6 further wedges longitudinally and the top half to be cut into 4. Place all the 10 wedge pieces on steaming rack and steam for 5 minutes or until slightly soft. Remove from heat.
- Heat 2 tbsp oil in wok. Add garlic, shrimps, chillies and sauté for a minute or until fragrant. Add eggplant and sauté for a minute. Add oyster sauce and stir to mix.
- Garnish with coriander and serve hot.

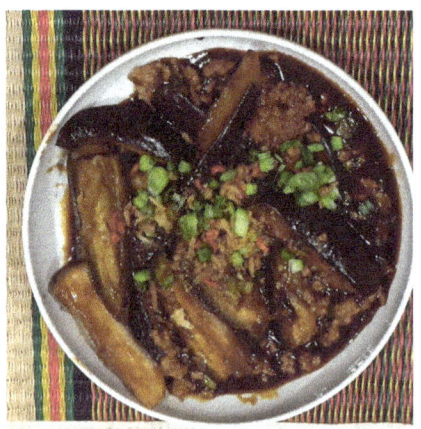

Variation: eggplant with mince instead of shrimp

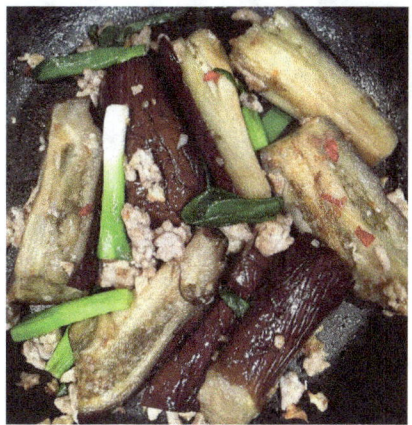

Variation: with turkey mince, chopped red chillies and 3" spring onions (scallions) cooked rather than as garnish.

SHRIMP OR PRAWN BEE HOON (RICE VERMICELLI)

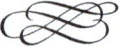

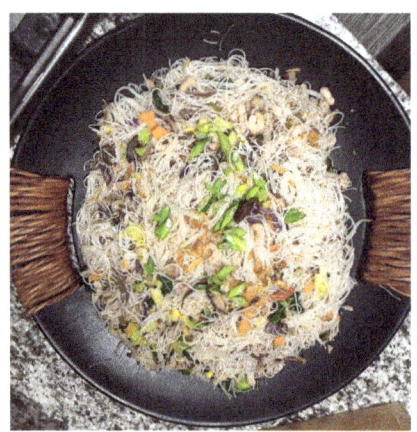

Bee hoon (mi fen in Mandarin, mai fun in Cantonese) is Hokkien for rice vermicelli. It's the classic snack when I was in school and even eaten as breakfast. It is also a standard party dish when you are growing up in Asia. It's notoriously difficult for the beginner because of the fast timing. **HOT TIP**: the bee hoon must not be overcooked (becoming clumpy or stuck together) or undercooked (rope-like). The moment the texture has changed from its raw thread-like state, you need to add the sauce mixture.

Serves 4-8 as party food or snacks

- 2 cloves garlic, chopped
- A whole packet of bee hoon (rice vermicelli) soaked in hot water for about half an hour or until soft
- ½ Chinese cabbage, chopped
- One third cup of wood ear (dried cloud ears) fungus soaked in hot water for 15 minutes
- 2 dried Chinese or shiitake mushrooms soaked in hot water for 15 minutes
- 1 cup of raw or cooked shrimps
- 1 carrot peeled into ribbons with vegetable peeler
- 1 handful spinach
- A splash of fish sauce
- A splash of sesame oil
- A splash of Shaoxing wine
- 1 tbsp rice bran oil or another healthy alternative
- 3 stalks of spring onions (the green part) sliced diagonally for garnish

1. Drain both the wood ear and Chinese mushrooms. Cut off the hard and woody stalks. Slice the mushrooms thinly. Drain the bee hoon.
2. Mix the sesame oil, fish sauce, wine with a quarter cup of water and set aside.
3. Heat oil in wok and add garlic, cabbage, mushrooms, shrimps. Sauté for 30 seconds or until fragrant.
4. Add the fish sauce mixture and replace lid on wok. Steam for 2 minutes.
5. Add bee hoon, carrot ribbons and spinach and further sauté for about a minute. This is the turning point, so watch out when it suddenly goes from raw to cooked. Switch off and remove from heat to prevent drying out. Add spring onion garnish and serve.

VEGAN BEE HOON

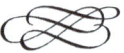

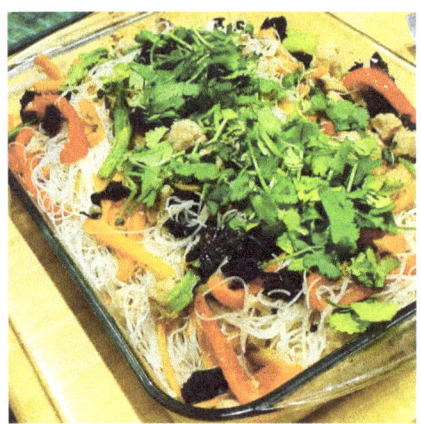

This is the vegan version, also colourful and tasty. **HOT TIP**: The beginner should start with this version before moving onto the shrimp version. In this version, you have to make vegetable stock, rather than the fish sauce combo.

Serves 4-8 as party food or snacks

- 2 cloves garlic, chopped

- A whole packet of rice vermicelli soaked in hot water for about half an hour or until soft
- ½ a cup of firm tofu, cut into cubes
- 1 red pepper, sliced
- 1 yellow pepper, sliced
- One third cup of wood ear (dried cloud ears) fungus soaked in hot water for 15 minutes
- 2 dried Chinese or shiitake mushrooms soaked in hot water for 15 minutes
- 1 cup of chopped mushrooms (any)
- 1 carrot cut into thin sticks/batons
- 1 handful spinach
- One third cup of vegetable stock
- A splash of sesame oil
- 1 tbsp rice bran oil or another healthy alternative
- ½ a bunch of coriander, torn roughly, for garnish

1. Drain both the wood ear and Chinese mushrooms. Cut off the hard and woody stalks. Slice the mushrooms thinly. Drain the bee hoon.
2. Heat oil in wok and add garlic, carrots, mushrooms, tofu. Sauté for 30 seconds or until fragrant.
3. Add the stock and replace lid on wok. Steam for 3 minutes. Open the lid and add bee hoon and further sauté for about a minute. This is the turning point, as per the shrimp version, so watch out when it suddenly goes from raw to cooked. Add the spinach and replace the lid so that it will wilt. Switch off the heat as when it has just cooked, it will start to dry up.
4. Add spring onion garnish and serve.

MY MUM'S KUNG PAO CHI TING
(KUNG PO CHICKEN)

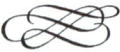

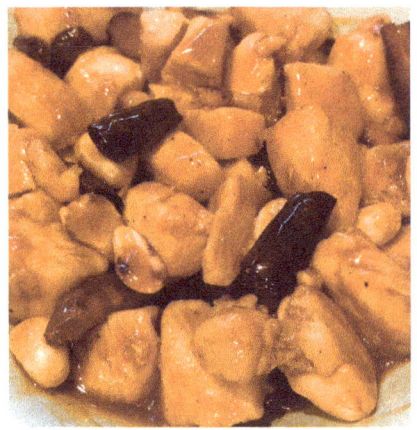

This is one of the first things I made as a fully grown adult trying to impress people with my cooking. You can substitute the chicken with pork, firm tofu, quorn pieces or turkey. The aim is to achieve that slick high shine finish. The dried chilli is so glossy it looks black. You can buy the dried chilli from any Chinese, Italian or Mediterranean (Middle-eastern) supermarkets. The most common question is why not use fresh red chilli. The reason is that dried chilli has a sundried, caramelised and smoky

30 CHINESE DINNERS

flavour. Also you want the big rectangular shapes for a bold visual effect. **HOT TIP:** don't use the beer snack form of ready-salted peanuts. They're too salty and oily thus ruining the delicate taste.

Serves 2-4

- 2 chicken breasts cut into cubes
- 2 cloves garlic, chopped finely
- A dash of Shaoxing wine
- Pepper
- Baking powder
- Approximately 4 or 5 whole large sundried chillies cut into 1 inch chunks
- 1 handful of raw unsalted peanuts (optional)
- 2 tbsp oil for frying like rice bran oil (or another healthy alternative)

For the sauce:

- 2 tbsp vinegar (any, but I used white wine vinegar)
- 2 tsp dark soy sauce
- A few drops of oyster sauce
- 2 tsp sugar or ½ tsp Stevia
- 1 tsp cornflour
- A quarter cup of water

1. Marinate the chicken in the garlic, wine, pepper and baking powder and leave for at least 4 hours or if you have no time or forgot, 20 minutes.
2. Dry roast the peanuts in a small frying pan for about 20 to 30 seconds. Watch carefully as they quickly burn. Remove form heat and keep aside.
3. Combine the dark soy sauce, oyster sauce, vinegar, sugar , water and flour in a cup and stir to mix well.
4. Rinse the dried chilli quickly to remove seeds but do not over

wash. They are not football boots and they will start to disintegrate like paper. Drain and dry on paper towels or tea towel.
5. Heat oil in wok until smoking. Add the dried chilli and stir for just 1-2 seconds as it burns quickly. Remove when brown and almost a glossy black. Set aside to cool.
6. Into the same oil in the wok, add chicken and roasted peanuts. Do not keep stirring or allow clumping. Allow meat to brown. This will take around 5 minutes. Toss with the spatula and spread over the whole wok area to ensure even cooking. Lower the flame.
7. Increase the fire. Spoon the sauce mixture into the wok, spoon by spoon and keep stirring.
8. When sauce is thickened, add the dried chilli. Stir quickly to mix it in.

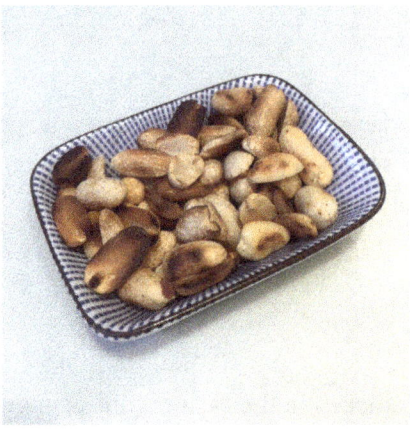

Hot tip: *You can pre-roast the peanuts just before cooking or on a different day.*

30 CHINESE DINNERS

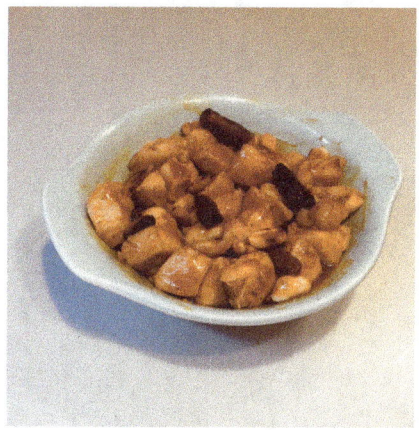

Aim for a slick high shine finish.

VEGAN CHOW MEIN

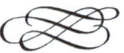

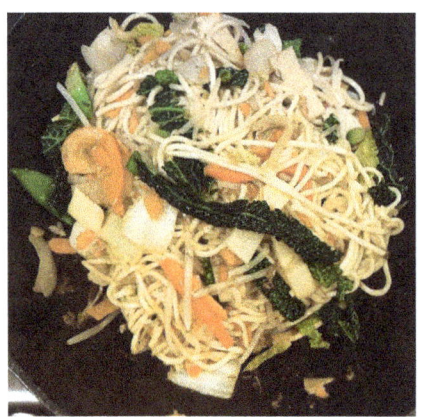

A handy quick healthy meal when there is nothing to eat but vegetables. This actually happened during the "2020 stockpiling and virus crisis". Now some of you may not "get" this business with the Shaoxing wine, but for that authentic Chinese restaurant taste, and especially so for vegan food, you need the wine and the chillies to amp up the dish and avoid that bland taste. This meal can be made in under 16 minutes. If you're me, probably 12 minutes. LOL.

Serves 2-4

- A packet of firm tofu, sliced and marinaded in black vinegar or Balsamic vinegar
- 2 cloves garlic, smashed
- 3 coils from a packet of wholewheat noodles
- Any finely sliced vegetables (eg kale, carrots, cabbage, mange tout are what's shown)
- A splash of soy sauce
- A splash of Shaoxing wine
- Red chillies finely sliced (optional)
- 2 tbsp rice bran oil for frying

1. Cook the noodles according to the packet. Remove from heat, drain and allow to cool slightly in the strainer.
2. Heat oil in wok and sauté garlic and tofu until fragrant.
3. Add all the vegetables at one go. Sauté for 1 minute. Add one third cup of water and replace lid to steam for 2 minutes.
4. Open lid and add the cooked noodles. Sauté to mix well for 1 minute. Add the soy sauce and wine.
5. Serve with red chillies as garnish (optional).

WOH TIP (POT STICKERS/ PAN STICKERS)

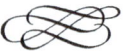

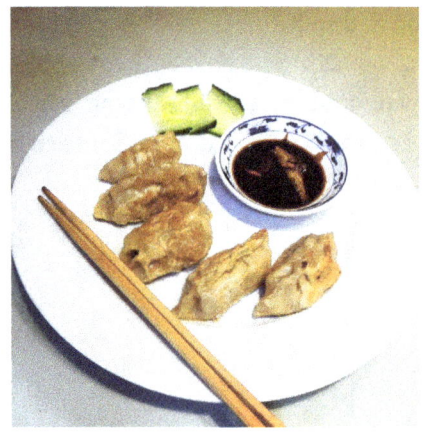

Versatile and popular, these can be served for a main meal or special occasions as a side dish. My children love them so they are perfect for after school snacks. The irony is despite the name, you have to make sure they do *not* stick to the pot/pan or else or Woh Tip dumplings will lose their "bottoms". LOL.

Serves 4-8

For the pastry

- 2 cups plain flour
- 3/4 cup water

For the filling

- 300g mince (pork, turkey, beef, lamb all work)
- 5 stalks Spring onions or scallions, finely chopped
- ½ a bunch of Chives (optional, finely chopped)
- 2 cloves garlic, minced finely
- 1 cup chopped leafy green vegetables eg pak choy, lettuce or Chinese cabbage
- 1 dsp sesame oil
- 2 dsp light soy sauce
- 2 tsp fresh ginger, minced finely

For the dip

- A bowl or dish of Chinking black Chinese vinegar (or Balsamic if you do not have black vinegar)
- A few strands of fresh ginger cut finely into threads
- Optional: red chillies, finely sliced

1. In a big mixing bowl, add water to the plain flour gradually and knead until it is a ball of dough. Cover and set aside while you make the filling.
2. Mix all the ingredients for the filling in another big bowl. Cover and set aside.
3. Tear off 1" balls of the dough and roll out each ball on a floured surface. When it is about 4-5" in diameter, place 1 dsp of the filling in the centre. Pull up the sides of the pastry like a tent to join at the top. Begin pleating 3 folds from the top to one end and another 3 folds from the bottom back to the top. Seal with drops of water if required or if the pastry is beginning to open. Each should look like a fat purse, and not a clam shell, with the pleated edges at the top.

I. NGEOW

4. Heat 2 tbsp of rice bran oil or another healthy alternative in a large wok. Add the dumplings 6-8 at a time (or how ever many can fit into the wok and still have gaps in between so that they are not touching each other). Turn the heat down to medium.
5. Once they are all golden brown, add a quarter cup of water to the wok and replace the lid. Turn the heat to high and steam for 4 minutes or until the wok is nearly dry and the water has disappeared.
6. Remove and repeat with batches of 6-8 dumplings at a time.
7. Serve with the black vinegar and ginger slivers. If you want you can also add finely sliced red chillies.

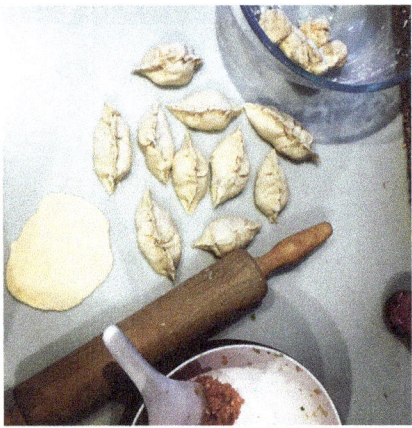

Tear off 1" balls of the dough and roll out each ball on a floured surface. When it is about 4-5" in diameter, place 1 dsp of the filling in the centre.

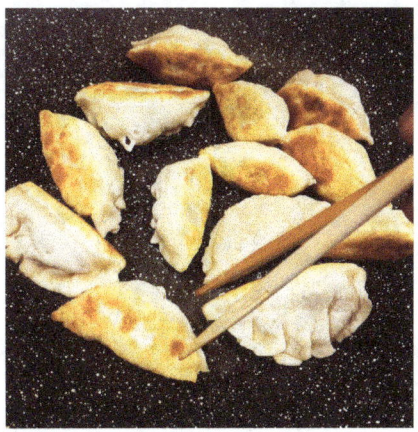

Keep turning them with a pair of wooden chopsticks to brown all sides and to make sure they are not sticking to each other or the pan.

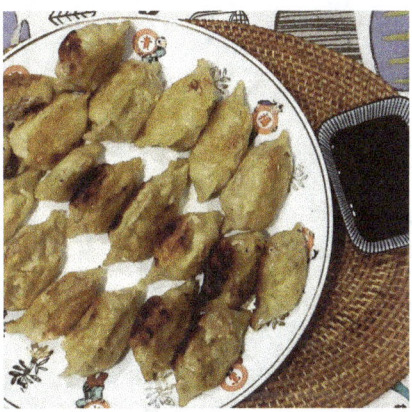

Serve with the black vinegar and ginger slivers. If you want you can also add finely sliced red chillies.

JUST PLAIN REGULAR LIGHT AND CRISPY TOFU

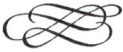

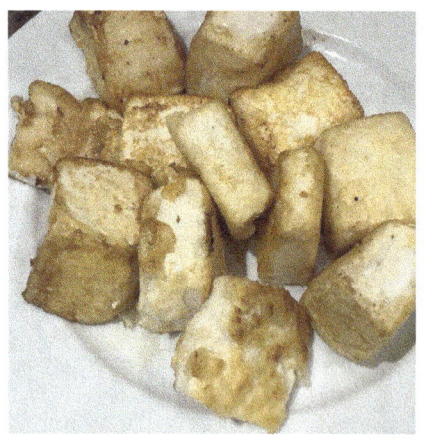

I say "just" tofu but it is so crispy and light you will not be requiring anything more than sweet chilli sauce.

Serves 2-4

- A packet of firm tofu, cut into large cubes
- 2-3 cloves garlic, minced
- A dash of salt

- 1 tbsp water if required
- 2 tbsp rice bran oil for frying or another healthy alternative

For the crispy batter

- 4 dsp wheat or plain flour
- 8 dsp tapioca flour or rice flour

1. Mix the first four ingredients in a large bowl and soak for 5-10 minutes while you prepare the batter.
2. Sift the 2 flours into a large bowl to combine them. Take the tofu out of the first mixture and coat with the flour evenly.
3. Heat oil in a wok until smoking. Lightly and quickly pan fry the tofu until golden brown. Remove and set on kitchen towel or paper towels.
4. Serve with sweet chilli sauce.

MY MUM'S MARMITE CHICKEN

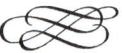

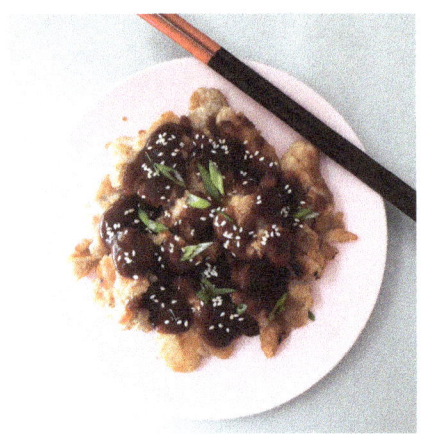

This is an unusual Anglo-Chinese meal for Marmite lovers. You can also use Vegemite if you like the Aussie equivalent. The idea for this dish is based on sweet and sour chicken because it's light and crispy chicken with a sauce. Be warned. It's a love or hate thing. If you hate Marmite, you should probably look away now.

Serves 2-4

- 1 tbsp Fab Four DIY marinade[1] (see back of book)
- 2 chicken breasts, cut into thin strips.

For the crispy batter

- 4 dsp wheat starch/flour
- 8 dsp tapioca starch/flour

For the marmite sauce

- 1 tbsp dark soy sauce
- 1-2 tsp marmite
- 1 tsp sugar or a sprinkle of Stevia
- 1 blob of squeezy honey
- 1 dash of pepper
- 1 dsp corn starch
- 2 tbsp water

For the garnish

- Toasted sesame seeds and/or spring onions (the green part) sliced diagonally.

1. Marinade the chicken for at least 4 hours or overnight. If you forgot or have no time, then at least 20 minutes while you make the sauce and the batter.
2. Optional: Preheat oven or air fryer to 190 deg C (375 deg F or gas mark 5)
3. Mix all of the sauce ingredients in a bowl.
4. Combine the two flours for the batter in a large and flattish dish such as an oven tray.
5. Put the chicken pieces into the flour mixture and coat well. Do not add water. Make sure it is dry and looks dry.
6. Heat 2 tbsp oil in a wok. Add the chicken pieces and lightly pan fry for 1-2 minutes to brown all sides. You can replace the

lid and move the wok to a smaller ring and carry on cooking until the chicken is fully cooked **OR** you can use this **HOT TIP**: remove par-cooked chicken and place in the air fryer or oven for about 12 minutes to prolong cooking time, while you make the sauce. This is to save time and oil frying.
7. Heat the sauce mixture in a small saucepan and keep stirring gently until it thickens. Switch off the fire.
8. Remove chicken from the oven or air fryer and put it back into the wok. Pour the sauce all over it. Stir in and mix well. Remove everything from wok and place on a serving plate or dish.
9. Sprinkle the toasted sesame seeds all over for garnish.

---

1. See Top 3 essential DIY marinades, sauces & pastes

HONG KONG CHINESE CHIVES OMELETTE

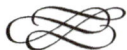

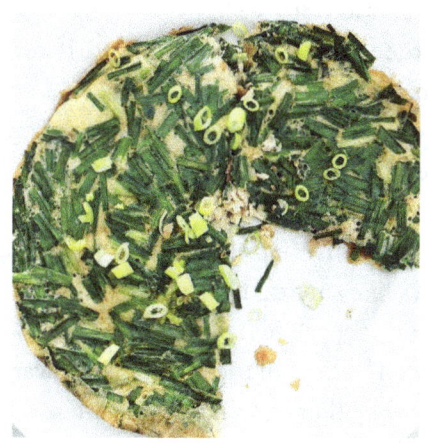

Chive talkin', ya tellin' me lies. Chinese chives are different from their Western equivalent. They are more pungent and have a coarser texture. In Chinese food, chives are used medicinally for blood-purifying. You can get them from a Chinese supermarket or a larger Western supermarket. This easy vegetarian meal is high protein and perfect for dim sum type situations, i.e. brunch. I love the strong garlicky flavour and taste of Chinese chives. A chilli sauce dip adds a proper finishing touch. Sweet does not really go with eggs, therefore, I prefer a hot garlicky chilli sauce rather than a sweet one, but this is down to your preference.

Serves 2-4

- 4 eggs
- 1 cup of Chinese chives cut to half an inch long
- 1 tsp fish sauce
- A few drops of Shaoxing wine
- 2 tsp corn starch
- 2 tsp water
- 2 tbsp rice bran oil or another healthy alternative
- 1 tbsp of chilli sauce to serve

1. In a large bowl, beat eggs. Add fish sauce, wine, chives, cornstarch, water and stir well.
2. Heat oil in large frying pan until smoking. If you do not have a large frying pan, use a small one and make 4 individual omelettes about 6" each in diameter. Pour the mixture in and fry the omelette until 80% puffy. Do not overcook or it will dry out and be rubbery.
3. Remove from heat. If you used a large frying pan, cut into four or more pieces like a pizza. If you used a small frying pan, remove each and repeat, just like making pancakes. The cooked ones can be kept in the oven to keep warm while you finish making the other individual omelettes.
4. Serve with chilli sauce.

SHRIMP AND CHINESE CABBAGE TAGLIATELLE

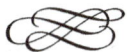

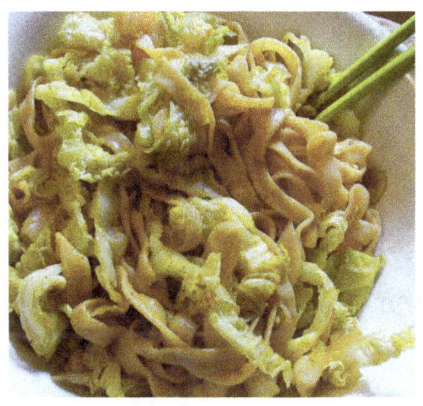

This is a modern fusion twist on a standard childhood meal which I have grown up with. I believe it is Cantonese in origin. Here, it is served with tagliatelle, which makes a change from rice. At first I thought only my family ate shrimp and cabbage. But later I noticed that when I went to my friends' homes for dinner or lunch, this humble dish came out too. The tagliatelle done Cantonese style still works as a very easy and tasty East-West meal.

Serves 2-4

I. NGEOW

- A cup of shrimps or little prawns, raw or cooked
- Famous Five marinade[1]
- 1 tsp of Shaoxing wine
- 1 Chinese cabbage
- Optional: 1 carrot cut finely into matchsticks
- 2 tbsp of rice bran oil or another healthy alternative

1. Mix the shrimps with the marinade in a bowl. Cook the tagliatelle according to the packet instructions, drain, rinse with cold tap water and leave aside.
2. Chop the cabbage into an inch long pieces and stop when you get to an inch from the stalk end.
3. Heat the oil in the wok until smoking. Add the shrimps and sauté for a minute or until fragrant. Add all the cabbage and (carrot if you are using carrot) and sauté for 1 minute. Add the tagliatelle, half a cup of water, stir and replace the lid of the wok. Allow to steam on high for 3 minutes.
4. Open the lid and add the Shaoxing wine. Stir to mix for about 30 seconds.
5. Serve with a side salad.

---

1. See *Top 3 essential DIY marinades, sauces & pastes* at the end of the book.

SINGAPORE PRAWN NOODLE SOUP (HEI MEE)

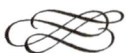

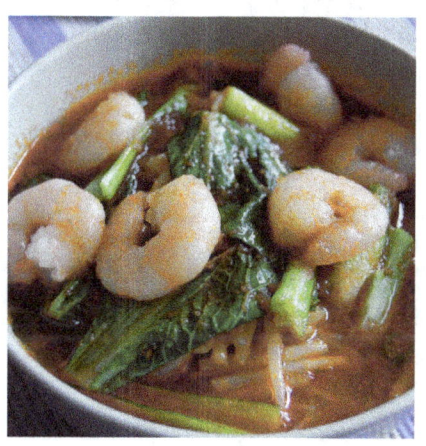

J ust to reiterate, I come from the Deep South so a lot of these dishes such as this one are not popular and not even available up north. Prawn mee is Hokkien in origin. Most of the time here is in making the broth which is sweet and sea-pungent, a particularly strong taste of home since I grew up next to the Straits. The actual assembly of the meal takes 5 minutes.

Serves 2-4

I. NGEOW

For the prawn broth (soup base)

- Heads and shells of 2 lbs or roughly 1 kg of raw prawns
- 3 lbs or roughly 1.5 kg of pork ribs chopped by the butcher into smaller pieces
- 8 cups of water
- 5 cloves garlic, peeled
- 5 white peppercorns
- 1 star anise
- 1 to 2 tsp of fish stock powder (optional)

For the noodle dish

- Prawns from the above heads and shells
- 1 bunch of water spinach (Kangkung, or ong choy) - if unavailable, substitute with baby spinach
- 2 cups of bean sprouts
- A splash of fish sauce
- 4-5 red chillies finely sliced
- Soy sauce in a small ceramic side dish (the size of a Petri dish)

1. Remove heads and shells of prawns and set aside prawns. You will need 5 prawns per serving.
2. Put all the broth ingredients into a slow cooker for about 4 hours.
3. Cook the noodles according to the packet instructions (usually 3 minutes), adding the raw prawns (5 per person or however many you'd like each person to have) midway, and in the final 2 minutes, adding the bean sprouts and spinach or water spinach and blanching them.
4. Drain the saucepan and serve noodles in bowls. **HOT TIP #1:** Arrange the 5 prawns last, on top of each bowl, in a fan-like shape. **HOT TIP #2:** Prawns are expensive, and you may like to cut costs. You can do the frugal thing and halve each prawn longitudinally. And wa-lah! From one prawn you get two.

5. Add the soup with a pork rib or two in each bowl.
6. Serve with the side dish of chillies floating in soy sauce. **HOT TIP #3:** If you make the broth in advance you can freeze it in batches and use it to make many more bowls of prawn noodle soup at some future point.

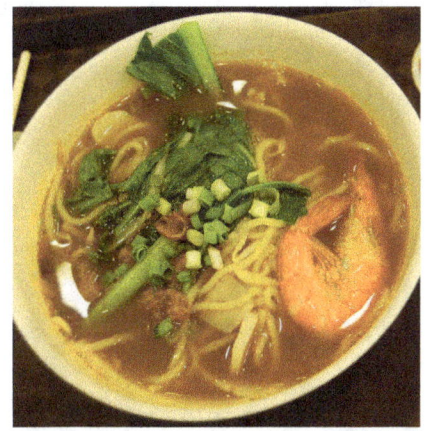

HAKKA CLAYPOT MINCE PORK AND TOFU

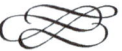

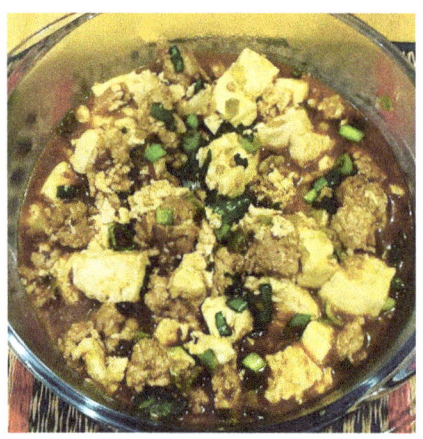

A hearty Hakka protein-rich meal that traditionally will set you up for a tough nomadic life and gruelling labour. Served with rice, pickled or fresh vegetables, it is nutritious, plain and comforting. The claypot preserves the earthy and wholesome flavours but if you don't have one, a cast iron casserole is just as good, which you can shove in the oven to keep warm or reheat. A normal saucepan or pot will achieve the basic job too. Incidentally, Hakka girls are known to be hardworking, no-nonsense and down to earth. Naturally this description does not apply to me, apart from the first adjective.

Serves 2-4

- 1 cup of minced pork
- 1 packet of medium firm or silken tofu, either is fine
- Marinade (see Fab Four in top 4 essential DIY marinades, sauces and pastes) for at least four hours if possible, if not a few minutes
- 2 tbsp rice bran oil or another healthy alternative
- White pepper
- Chopped coriander, spring onion (scallions) and crumbed salted fish (optional) for garnish

For the sauce

- Half a cup of water
- 1 tsp oyster sauce
- 2 tsp cornflour
- A few drops of Shaoxing wine

1. Put all the sauce ingredients in a jug and stir to mix well.
2. Roughly chop up the tofu into large cubes.
3. Heat oil in wok. When hot, add the mince pork and break it up so it does not clump together. Sauté for about 2 minutes.
4. Add tofu and sauté for another 2 minutes. Do not stir like an earthquake or the tofu shapes will be destroyed and turn into scrambled egg. Go easy and stir by overturning the pieces of mince and tofu gently and without cutting anything up. This is why you need a wide, very flat-edged spatula and not a wooden spoon. The thickness of the wooden spoon's lip will start to scramble the cubes.
5. Add a quarter cup of water and cover with the wok lid to steam for 2 minutes.

6. Open the lid. Pour the sauce over and allow to thicken. Again, stir a little to quicken the thickening process but do not over stir.
7. Remove from heat and serve with garnish with pickles, spinach and lettuce salad for a low carb option or with rice.

CHICKEN CHOW MEIN

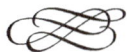

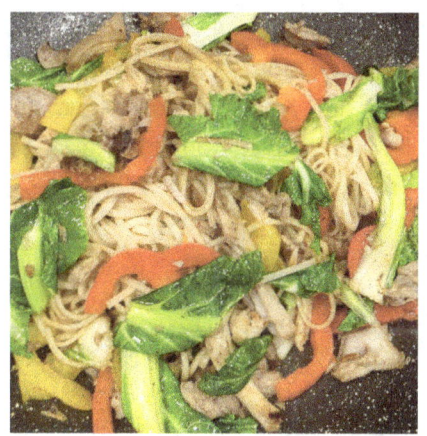

This is a classic simple healthy meal with that traditional Chinese restaurant taste but non-greasy.

Serves 2-4

- 2 cups of raw chicken, finely sliced
- 3 coils from a packet of wholewheat noodles
- Marinade (see Fab Four in top 3 essential DIY marinades,

I. NGEOW

sauces and pastes) for at least four hours if possible, if not a few minutes
- Green leafy vegetables (sweetheart cabbage or cauliflower leaves as shown)
- 2 tbsp rice bran oil or another healthy alternative
- 1 red bell pepper, sliced
- 1 yellow bell pepper, sliced
- A dash of white pepper
- Chopped coriander and spring onion (scallions) for garnish (optional)

1. Marinade the chicken for at least 4 hours if possible or if you forgot, a few minutes will do while you cook the noodles.
2. Cook the noodles according to the packet. Remove from heat, drain and allow to cool slightly in the strainer.
3. Heat oil in wok and sauté chicken until fragrant.
4. Add all the vegetables at one go. Sauté for 1 minute. Add one third cup of water and replace lid to steam for 2 minutes.
5. Open lid and add the cooked noodles. Sauté to mix well for 1 minute.
6. Serve with red chillies as garnish (optional).

HOT TIP: You can cheat by using cooked leftover chicken, eg roast chicken.

1. Debone and skin the chicken until you get about 2 cups' worth of meat.
2. As there is no marinade, mix the sauce in a separate jug consisting of half a cup of water, a tsp of cornflour, a splash of Shaoxing wine, 1 dsp oyster sauce. Stir.
3. Sauté 1 clove of chopped garlic (or minced garlic from a jar), add the roast chicken and the vegetables all at one go and sauté for 2 minutes. Add the sauce mixture. Replace the lid and steam for 2 min.
4. Open lid and add the cooked noodles. Mix well for 1 minute.

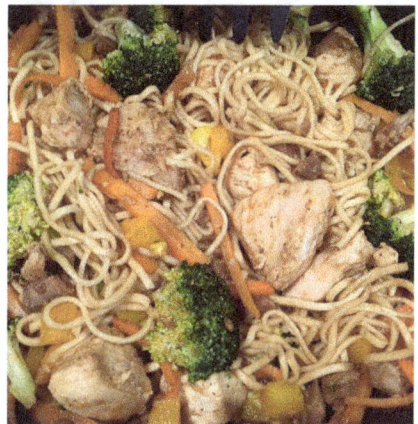

Variation: using chunkier and juicier pieces of chicken and broccoli for that "Chinese takeaway" authenticity.

THREE MUSHROOM TOFU

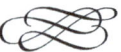

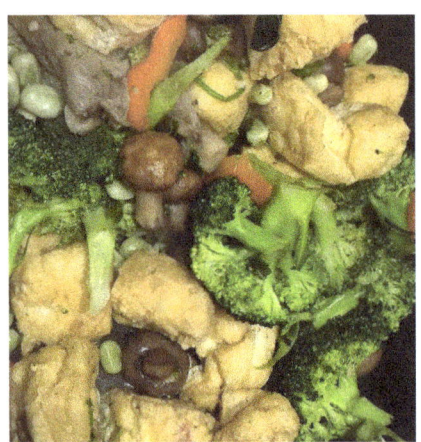

I rarely cook this as no one in the family likes mushrooms but me. If you use silken or soft tofu, it will easily collapse and crumble into something that is like custard so it is really not for this dish. Use tofu that is already pre-cooked or pre-fried to save time. It also improves the texture and density because the pre-cooked tofu is chunky and meaty in texture like little sponges, and this makes it hold the flavours better.

Serves 4

- 1 packet of pre-cooked or fried tofu, cut into cubes
- 1 tbsp rice bran oil or another healthy alternative
- 3 garlic cloves, crushed
- 25g (1 oz) Chinese dried mushrooms (shiitake) pre-soaked in hot water for at least 20 minutes
- Wood ear black fungus, soaked in hot water for at least 20 minutes, sliced into big pieces.
- One third cup fresh close cup or button mushrooms, sliced thickly
- 1 carrot cut into thin matchsticks
- A splash of light soy sauce
- A splash of Shaoxing wine
- 1 tbsp oyster sauce
- 1 stalk of scallions/spring onions, thinly sliced for garnish
- Dried salted fish crumbs (optional) for garnish

1. Drain the Chinese mushrooms through a sieve and keep the water from soaking for cooking rice or making soups. Squeeze the mushrooms dry with fingers. Slice thinly and discard the hard stalks.
2. Use one third cup of the water from soaking. Add 1 dsp cornflour, the light soy sauce, Shaoxing wine, oyster sauce and stir to dissolve the cornflour.
3. Heat the oil in the wok until slightly smoking. Add the garlic and sauté for a few seconds until fragrant. Add all the vegetables and tofu except the scallions/spring onions. Sauté until well mixed for a few seconds more.
4. Pour in the water mixed with cornflour. Bring to a boil. Turn the heat down. Keep stirring until the sauce thickens. Mix in the scallions/spring onions and serve on its own or with a plate of sliced red chillies.

Hot tip: A light sprinkle of dried salted fish crumbs will lend an authentic finishing touch.

AUBERGINE (EGGPLANT) THAI RED CURRY AND CAULIFLOWER RICE

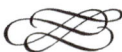

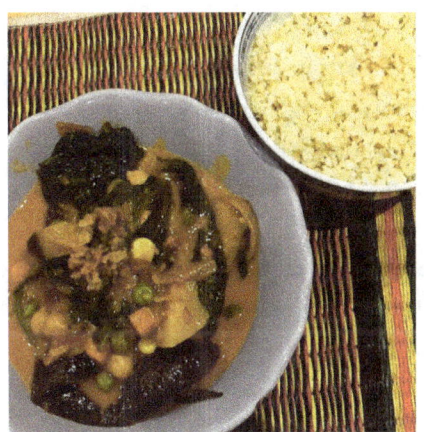

This is a quick low carb meal for those days when you are feeling terrible. It will instantly refresh you. A light vegetarian curry can be revitalising. You don't need to go to a yoga and spa weekend. Realistically, it will only take about 20 minutes. **HOT TIP:** save the leftover tinned pineapple juice and chunks in the fridge as you can use it another day in another meal (sweet and sour meatballs).

Serves 2-3

- 1 aubergine
- 1 cauliflower
- 1 cup of frozen vegetables (eg with peas, carrots and baby corn)
- 1 bunch of spinach

For the curry

- 2 tbsp red curry paste
- 1 tin of coconut milk/cream
- 4 kaffir lime leaves, ripped
- Famous Five paste[1]
- 1 tbsp sugar or half tsp Stevia
- 3 tbsp pineapple juice
- Half a cup of tinned pineapple cubes
- Half a cup of holy or sweet basil leaves, ripped
- 1 large red chilli finely sliced for garnish.
- 2 tbsp rice bran oil or another healthy alternative

1. Cut the aubergine or eggplant into cross sectioned first, then longitudinally. The top half into 3 and the bottom, or the bigger half, into 4.
2. Pluck off the cauliflower florets by hand and blitz them in a food processor until they appear like crumbs. Put in a large ceramic bowl.
3. Steam in a rack for 5 minutes or until soft. Remove from heat.
4. Heat oil in a wok until hot. Add garlic and brown it until fragrant. Lower heat. Add curry paste, lime leaves and aubergine and sauté on medium for about 2 minutes or until fragrant.
5. Add aubergine and all the frozen vegetables . Sauté for 2 minutes.
6. Add coconut milk and bring to boil. Reduce heat to low and

add fish sauce, sugar or Stevia, pineapple juice and pieces. Replace lid. Simmer for 4 minutes.
7. While it's simmering, add a little water (half a cup, say) to the bowl containing the cauliflower crumbs. Microwave for 5 minutes on high.
8. Switch off the fire. Open wok lid and add spinach leaves. Replace lid to wilt them for a few seconds while you remove the cauliflower from the microwave. Remove curry from heat, add the garnish and the holy basil or sweet basil leaves. Serve with the hot cauliflower rice.

---

1. See *Top 3 essential DIY marinades, sauces and pastes* at the end of the book

MY DAUGHTER'S 5-INGREDIENT CHICKEN IN 10 MINUTES

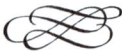

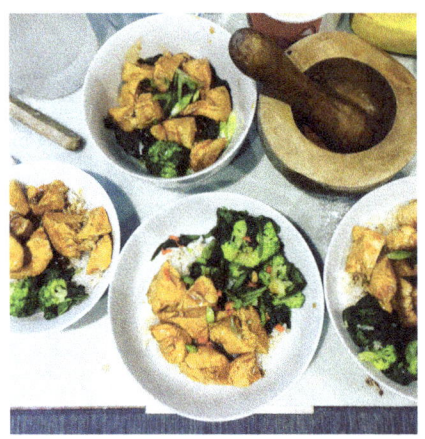

At the time of writing, my daughter was 9 and made this simple meal all by herself for a light summer dinner outside. She said she'd like to cook for the family and will "just improvise and surprise me". I was so thrilled I didn't care what she was making. OK it was fantastic. You're been warned: it's child's play so go have fun.

Serves 2-4

- 2-3 chicken breasts cut into large chunks
- 2 cloves of garlic, finely minced
- 1 tbsp soy sauce
- 1 tbsp Chinese cooking wine
- A squirt of squeezy honey
- 2 tsp cornflour
- 2 tbsp rice bran oil for frying, or another healthy alternative
- Spring onion (scallions), the green part only, thinly-shredded into slivers
- 1 red chilli, finely-sliced, as garnish (optional)

1. Heat oil in wok until hot. Add the chicken and the garlic and sauté for 3 minutes until brown and fragrant. Add a quarter cup of water and shut the wok lid to steam for about 5 minutes. Adjust the timing according the size of the chicken chunks (the bigger, the longer the steaming time and more water you need to add).
2. Make the sauce by mixing the soy sauce, honey, cooking wine, cornflour and a third cup of water in a small jug or bowl. Stir well to avoid lumps.
3. Open the lid of the wok. Sauté again for a few seconds to check the chicken is cooked. Pour in the sauce mixture from the jug and keep stirring until the sauce thickens. Add the spring onions and mix in quickly.
4. Serve hot with steamed broccoli, blanched spinach and hot steaming brown rice. **HOT TIP #1:** sprinkle toasted flaked almonds to the spinach for a modern and fragrant twist. **HOT TIP #2:** Cook the rice in the rice cooker *before* you cook the chicken, because that will take 10-12 minutes. **HOT TIP #3:** Boil the broccoli and blanch the spinach during the 5 minutes of steaming the chicken. Wa-lah! All hot and ready at the same time. A perfectly-timed meal in 10 minutes. No, really.

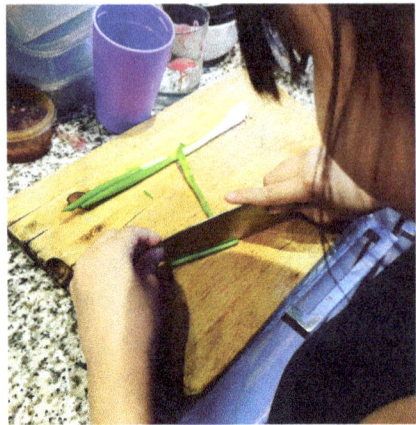

Her idea was to cut the green part of the spring onions (scallions) into slivers.

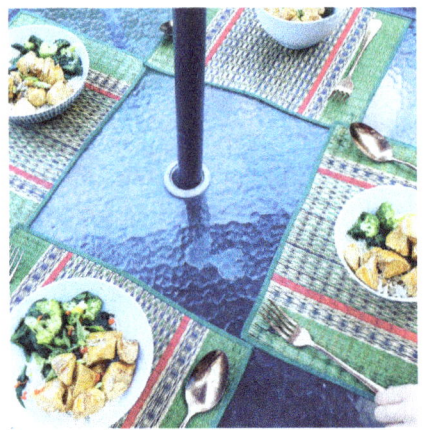

Perfect for a light summer evening family meal outside.

MY GRANNY'S MINCED PORK WITH NOODLES (HAKKA MEIN)

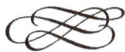

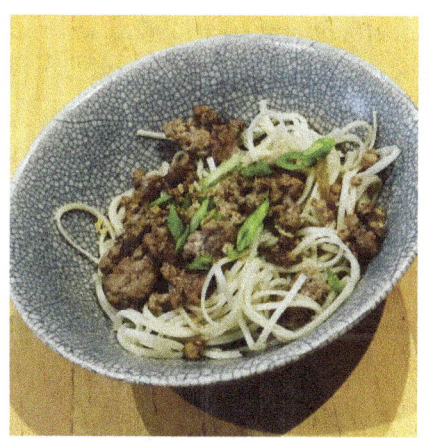

This is what my granny used to call the Hakka spaghetti bolognese. Apart from the lack of bolognese sauce, I would say it is similar. The pork mince has the exact same treatment as for the claypot dish and pretty much any Hakka dish involving pork mince. Thanks to Marco Polo you can use spaghetti or linguine for the medium (not the fine) egg noodles, and balsamic for black vinegar. If you are vegetarian you may like to substitute the mince with quorn or vegetarian mince.

I. NGEOW

Serves 2-4

- 1 cup of minced pork
- 2-3 cups of noodles, spaghetti or linguine
- Marinade (see Fab Four in top 4 essential DIY marinades, sauces and pastes) for at least four hours if possible, if not a few minutes
- 2 tbsp rice bran oil or another healthy alternative
- White pepper
- A few drops of black vinegar such as Chinkiang black vinegar or balsamic
- A splash of sesame oil
- Chopped coriander , finely sliced red chilli and spring onion (scallions) for garnish

1. Cook the spaghetti, linguine or noodles according to the packet instructions. Drain and rinse with cold water to stop overcooking and sticking.
2. Heat oil in wok until hot. Sauté the pork mince for 3 minutes until cooked. Add the cooked spaghetti, linguine or noodles and mix well. Add a splash of sesame oil to stop them sticking.
3. Add a few drops of black vinegar to a tbsp of water and add to the wok. Stir and serve with the garnish.

CHICKEN MACARONI SOUP (SLOW COOKER)

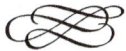

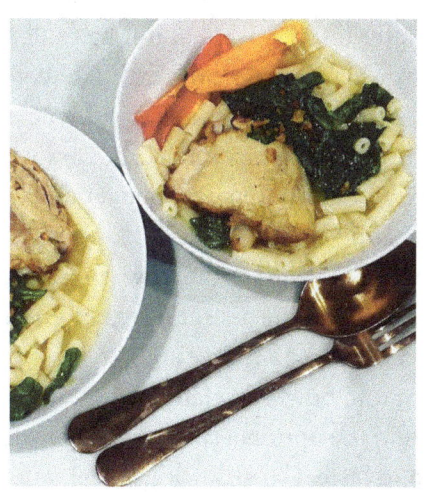

I grew up eating this comfort meal as a child and now my children love it and often ask for it. This is especially good when you are ill or have had dental treatment because it's hydrating and it's soft food. The best thing is that it is so simple and with the slow cooker you just switch it on while you do something else. It's a real time-saver for a family. I don't know if it's also come from Marco Polo because it's another traditional Chinese meal with pasta in it.

I. NGEOW

Serves 2-4

- 4 chicken thighs, skinless and with all visible fat removed
- 2 cups of macaroni
- A thumb-size of ginger, sliced
- 2 carrots, cut into small cubes, about half inch
- A bunch of spinach (optional)
- 1 tbsp dried crispy fried shallots for garnish
- 1 stalk of spring onion (scallions) finely sliced for garnish
- 1 fish stock cube (optional)
- Ground white pepper
- Spraying oil

1. Spray the oil into a pan or in the slow cooker, sear or brown the chicken all over. Start the slow cooker and set it for 3 hours. Pour water into it such that it is half full.
2. Set your phone alarm, or some other timer, to go off in 2 hours' time (from the start of the slow cooking) to add the carrots and the optional stock cube. The carrots would therefore have an hour in the slow cooker and everybody will finish cooking at the same time.
3. During the last 15 minutes of the slow cooking, cook the macaroni according to the packet instruction. Drain and rinse under the cold tap to stop it sticking.
4. Dish macaroni into bowls and ladle out the soup, carrots and the chicken. Add the optional spinach. Grind white pepper onto the soup to taste. Garnish with spring onion (scallions) and the dried crispy fried shallots.

SWEET AND SOUR MEATBALLS (OR FISH)

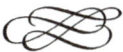

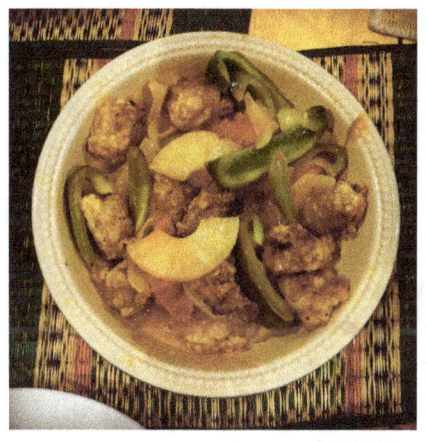

Hello! Another Chinese restaurant classic. Sweet and sour is Cantonese in origin, as are most dishes with the word "sour" such as hot and sour soup. If you come from the south in Malaysia, like I have, it is pretty much a restaurant dish and not as common at home. Johor, where I was born, is the home of pineapple, rubber and coffee plantations. You may also like to substitute the pork with fish. My son prefers the pork option.

Sweet and sour fish was very popular in my childhood home as my dad is very fond of pineapple. It is not as quick as the other recipes in this book because of the two-step process, i.e. making the battered fish then the sauce.

HOT TIP #1: If you have been paying attention, then you would have seen that to make Thai red curry sauce (for the aubergine Thai red curry) we required pineapple juice and chunks. You may now up-cycle the leftovers from the tin which you have hopefully kept aside in the fridge.

HOT TIP #2: I am being controversial here but I am making this dish a healthy alternative. Instead of deep frying the battered meatballs or fish chunks, I will shallow fry to brown it and then transfer the meatballs or fish to the air fryer or an oven if you do not have an air fryer. It will still be very tasty but will be less greasy and better for you. How about that?

Serves 2-4

- 1 kg or about 2 lbs of chunky white fish such as cod or halibut cut into 1" chunks OR minced pork rolled into 2" "lion's head" balls
- 1 large green pepper quartered into wedges
- 1 large tomato quartered into wedges
- 1 large onion quartered into wedges
- 1 tin of pineapple chunks in juice
- 2 tbsp rice bran oil

For the batter

- ¼ cup corn flour
- 2 cups plain flour
- 2 tablespoons rice bran oil
- 4 teaspoons baking powder
- A pinch of salt

- A pinch of chilli powder
- About 2 cups of water

For the sweet and sour sauce

- ½ tbsp sugar or ½ tsp Stevia
- ½ cup pineapple juice
- 2 tbsp ketchup
- 2 tablespoons corn flour

1. Preheat air fryer or oven if you have no air fryer to 90 deg C or 375 deg F.
2. Dry the fish with kitchen paper if it's dripping wet or has been defrosted. Put the ¼ cup corn flour in a large plate and coat the fish in it.
3. Put the rest of the batter ingredients except the oil and water in a large bowl and mix well. Gradually add water and with a hand whisk or electric hand mixer, beat until the batter is smooth and without lumps. It should have the consistency of freshly-mixed cement (if you've ever poured concrete) i.e. not too thick or too thin. To test this, turn the bowl almost upside down. If the batter is flowing slowly, it's the correct consistency. If it's fast flowing, it's too runny and if it doesn't flow at all, it's actually concrete.
4. Pour the batter over the fish chunks or meatballs and coat thoroughly.
5. Heat 2 tbsp of oil in a frying pan or wok. Fry the chunks lightly for about 2 minutes to brown both sides. Remove and place in air fryer or oven for 18 minutes. While it is in the air fryer or oven, make the sauce.
6. Put all the ingredients of the sauce into a jug and mix well.
7. Heat 2 tbsp oil in a wok or saucepan. When hot, add the onions, green pepper, pineapple and tomato and sauté for 3 minutes. Add the sauce mixture from the jug and keep stirring until the sauce thickens. Switch off the heat.

8. Remove the fish chunks or meat balls from the air fryer or oven and set onto a serving plate. Pour the sauce with the vegetables all over the fish or meatballs and serve with rice.

VARIATION: SWEET AND SOUR CHICKEN (CHIU CHOW OR TEOCHEW STYLE) I.E. WITHOUT PINEAPPLE

Serves 2-4

If there's no pineapple or pineapple juice in the house, you can still make sweet and sour sauce, for example this sweet and sour chicken.

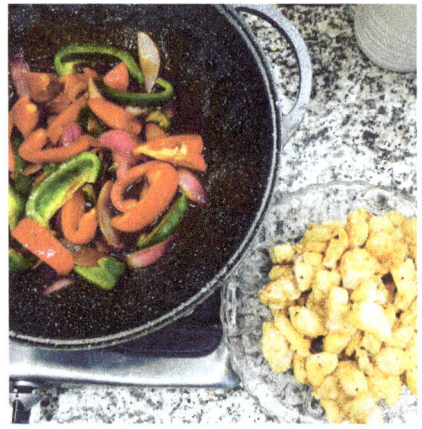

Before combining the vegetables, sauce and the cubes of chicken

Cut 2 chicken breasts up into cubes[1], batter and cook all as per the recipe for meatballs or cod above. Chop onions, green pepper, yellow pepper and tomatoes.

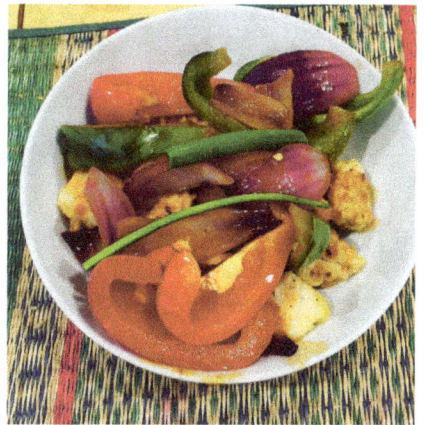

After combining chicken, sauce and vegetables. Optional: use long thin shreds of the green part of spring onions (scallions) for garnish.

For the sweet and sour sauce (without pineapple)

- 2 tbsp ketchup
- A few drops of light soy sauce
- A splash of sesame oil
- 1½ to 2 tbsp white wine vinegar or rice wine vinegar
- 1 dsp sugar or ½ tsp Stevia
- 3 tsp cornflour
- ½ cup water

1. Put all the ingredients of the sauce into a jug and mix well.
2. Heat 2 tbsp oil in a wok or saucepan. When hot, add the onions, green pepper, yellow pepper and tomato and sauté for 3 minutes. Add the sauce mixture from the jug and keep stirring until the sauce thickens. Switch off the heat.
3. Set the chicken onto a serving plate. Pour the sauce with the vegetables all over the chicken and serve with rice.

---

1. My daughter calls these "chicken popcorn" — that should give you an idea of the size.

STEAMED SEABASS IN 15 MINUTES

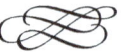

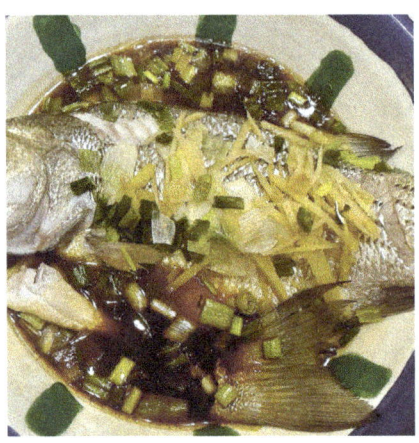

Traditionally you would steam and serve the entire fish whole, top to tail. Get the scaled and cleaned up version from the fishmongers. You do not turn the fish upside down. If you believe the old wives' tales, the superstition is that it's bad luck and that your ship will capsize. Therefore after you eat one side, you should instead lift the vertebrae off to expose the other side.

Serves 2

- 1 seabass
- A thumb-sized knob of ginger, finely sliced
- Steaming plate and rack
- Crumbed dried salted fish and/or crispy fried garlic for garnish

For the dressing

- 2 tbsp Shaoxing wine
- 1 tbsp sesame oil
- A cup of coriander, finely chopped
- ½ tsp sugar or a pinch of Stevia
- 1 dsp soya sauce

1. Score the fish in diagonals on both sides, four scores per side. Put some slices of ginger onto the steaming plate and the fish onto it. Put the rest of the ginger slices on the fish.
2. Fill the wok to a third with water. Place the steaming rack into it, and then the plate of fish. Steam for 15 minutes or until tender and the juices are filling up on the plate. Remove the steaming plate from the wok carefully.
3. Put all the dressing ingredients into a large jug and stir vigorously with chopsticks. Transfer the fish and juices from the steaming plate onto a large oval serving dish and pour the dressing over. Sprinkle the salted fish and/or crispy fried garlic over for the garnish.
4. Serve with rice and a vegetable dish such as kai lan, pak choy, or choy sum sauté in garlic.

CRISPY ROAST DUCK WITH PANCAKES

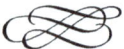

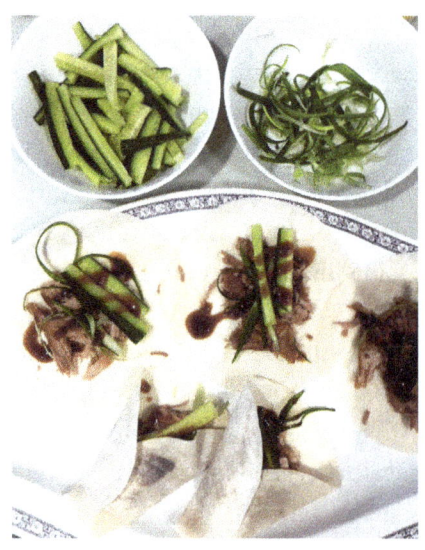

A wonderful cheat's meal that has gone from special occasion to any occasion, including weekends and lunch. This is a quicker method because as a very busy mother I am trying to save time and not do things the hard way.

Serves 4-6

30 CHINESE DINNERS

- 4 duck breasts, thighs or 2 of each
- 1 cucumber cut into thin matchsticks
- A bunch of spring onion, shredded
- Hoisin sauce from the squeezy bottle
- Sriracha chilli sauce (optional) from the squeezy bottle
- A packet of Chinese pancakes*

For the marinade

- 1 tsp garlic, finely chopped
- 1 tsp ginger, finely chopped
- 2 tsp five spice powder
- A squirt of honey from the squeezy bottle
- 1 splash of soy sauce
- A dash of white pepper

1. If using duck breasts score them in a criss crossing style with an inch spacing. Mix the marinade ingredients into a large bowl. Rub into the cuts with the marinade and leave the duck breasts for a few hours or overnight if possible. If not using breasts, just marinade them.
2. Switch on the grill to full and grill both sides of the breasts for 3 minutes each. Switch off the grill.
3. Preheat oven to 190 deg C or 375 deg F.
4. While it's heating up prepare the vegetables by thinly cutting the cucumber and shredding the spring onions. **HOT TIP #1**: To get the spring onions or scallions curly, soak them in water after shredding.
5. Place the pre-grilled duck in the oven and roast for 25-30 minutes or until golden brown.
6. Remove from oven and shred the duck meat with two forks. Serve on a large serving dish.
7. The children or your guests can all DIY and wrap their own duck individual pancakes. The pancake is placed on a flat plate. If you are using show-bought pancakes, make sure they

are microwaved for 30 seconds to a minute first. Put the duck, the cucumber and the spring onion on the pancake. Drizzle with the hoisin sauce and wrap or roll like a swaddle or blanket. Sides, bottom, top.

*HOT TIP #2: you can make your own pancakes rather than use the shop-bought one but it does add another layer of work (see below). If you need to cut the labour and time due to starving impatient children, then please stick with the shop-bought pancakes and don't feel guilty. They are getting roast duck, are they not?

Making your own pancakes

Mix 150 g of plain flour with half a cup of hot water and a pinch of salt. Mix well until it forms a dough. Allow to cool down slightly and knead for 5-10 minutes. Break the big ball of dough up into 2" diameter balls. Roll out with a rolling pin to thin circles each about 6-8" in diameter. Spray oil onto a flat frying pan. Fry both sides of each pancake just like a regular pancake. Remove from heat and allow a few minutes for handling and rolling up.

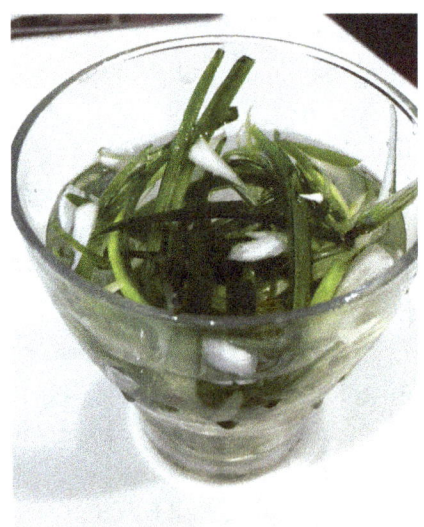

Soak the spring onions in water after shredding to get them curly.

30 CHINESE DINNERS

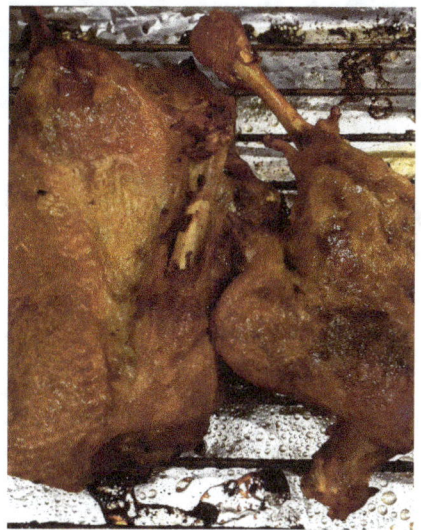

Pre-oven grilling will make the skin crispy and appear to "pop off".

BLANCHED PAK CHOY

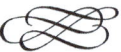

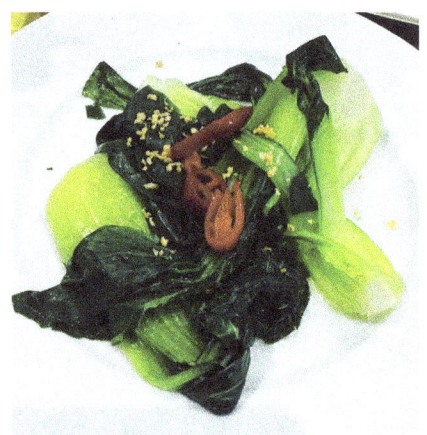

Pak choy (bok choy, pak choi, bai cai etc) is an easy side dish but it can be a main if paired with steamed chicken or tofu if you are doing low carb, or with rice and another dish. It is perfectly juicy and tasty on its own. As it is a cruciferous vegetable, it is high in anti-oxidants and minerals such as iron, calcium and zinc.

Serves 2-4

- 1 tsp of the Holy Trinity[1] paste
- 3 or 4 pak choy
- 1 tsp bicarbonate of soda
- 1 tbsp of sesame oil
- ½ tbsp of soy sauce
- Crispy fried garlic crumbs and a finely sliced red large chilli for garnish
- 2 tbsp oil for frying

- Heat the oil in a frying pan and sauté the paste until fragrant. Remove from pan. Mix the oil, paste and soy sauce in a small jug to make the dressing.
- Heat a large saucepan or a wok of water until it's boiling. Quarter the pak choy longitudinally. Add the pak choy and bicarbonate of soda and leave for 2 minutes. Switch off the heat and leave the pak choy in there for another minute. Remove and set on serving dish.
- Pour the dressing over and garnish with the crispy fried garlic crumbs and sliced red chilli. **HOT TIP #1:** if you don't have a fresh red chilli, you can use sliced red jalapeños from a jar. They work just as well. **HOT TIP #2:** You can make the dressing in advance and store it in the fridge. Consequently, if you made too much of the dressing, also just store it in the fridge for another salad or vegetable dish at some future point. This is a top hack for any vegetarian meal. Create a dressing and you create a world.

---

1. See *Top 3 essential DIY marinades, sauces & pastes* at the end of the book.

BEEF HOR FUN (FLAT RICE NOODLES)

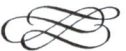

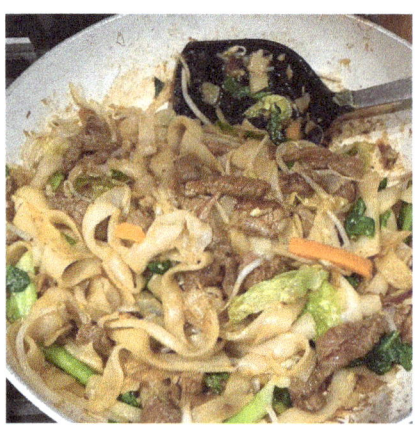

This Cantonese dish (full name: gon chow ngao hor fun) is a dry hor fun without gravy or soup. It is not to be confused with the soup hor fun or the sar hor fun which has the gloopy gravy. My favourite is the Ipoh sar hor fun as I love the thick slippery gravy. This beef hor fun is a good starter. It is a classic street food choice.

The actual cooking time is under 8 minutes approximately. Most of the time is in the preparation. **HOT TIP:** to save prep time, you can use quarter of a bag of the instant stir-fry green vegetable mix from the supermarket. It will contain all the usual pre-prepared suspects eg carrots, greens, bean sprouts etc.

Once lined up, all the ingredients are ready to go. But we warned: this is a tricky dish for the novice. I was caught myself a couple of times when I took my eye off the wok for a minute. There is a crucial turning point when it goes from cooked to overcooked. Practice is key. Overcooked noodles turn hard and rubbery from soft and silky.

Serves 2

- 1 cup of steak very thinly sliced across the grain
- 3 stalks of spring onions (scallions)
- 1 packet (around 3 cups) of fresh sa hor fun or dried if you can't get the fresh version
- 1-2 cups of bean sprouts
- 1 carrot thinly sliced (optional)
- 1 handful of green leafy vegetables, eg spinach, spring greens, sweetheart cabbage etc (optional) all sliced thinly
- Sliced green chillies or jalapeños from jar for garnish
- 2 tbsp rice bran oil for frying or another healthy alternative

For the marinade

- The fab 4
- ½ tsp cornflour
- 1 tbsp water

For the sauce

- 1 tsp cornflour
- 3 tbsp water
- 1 tbsp dark soy sauce

- ½ tsp sugar or a pinch of Stevia

1. Marinade the beef and chill in fridge overnight or for at least a few hours.
2. If using dried hor fun, soak in a big bowl of hot water for 20 minutes and then rinse in cold to stop the strands sticking. Loosen and separate as you are rinsing it. If using fresh hor fun, microwave in a big bowl in cycles of 30 seconds, taking out in between cycles to loosen and to separate the strands. This step is important to prevent clumping.
3. Cut the green part from the white of spring onions and set aside separately. Smash down the white part with the knife handle.
4. Spray oil onto a flat frying pan, heat it to smoking and sear the beef for 1 to 2 minutes. Do not overcook as it will be very tough. If in doubt, just sear for 1 minute and switch off. Remove from heat and keep aside.
5. Heat oil in wok until smoking. Add the white spring onions. Sauté for a minute or until fragrant. Add the vegetables if you are using them and sauté for 2 minutes.
6. Add the noodles and the sauce and sauté for 1-2 minutes or until it has softened and turned translucent. Immediately add the beansprouts, green part of the spring onions and the beef and keep stirring for another 1 minute maximum. Switch off heat, remove and serve hot.

5-INGREDIENT SHRIMP AND GREEN BEANS IN 10 MINUTES

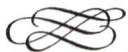

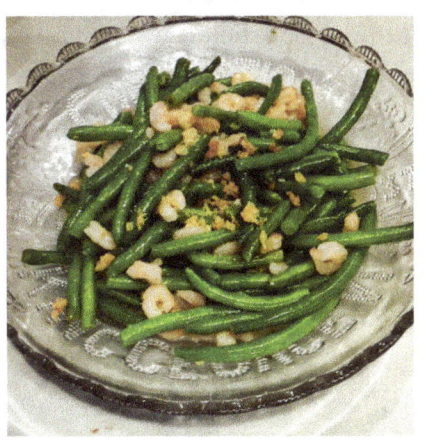

A low carb 5-ingredient meal in 10 minutes is great news when you are short of time or have come home and there's nothing ready to eat. This is where you would use frozen prawns (shrimps) and frozen beans. **HOT TIP:** always keep these in your freezer to rustle up an almost instant meal that is quicker than calling for a takeaway.

Serves 2-4

I. NGEOW

- 1 cup of frozen prawns (shrimps)
- 2 cups of frozen beans, or fresh if you have fresh
- 2 cloves of garlic, sliced finely
- 2 tbsp rice bran oil for frying or another healthy alternative
- 1 splash of Shaoxing wine

1. Heat oil in wok until hot. Put the garlic, prawns and the beans in and sauté for 2-3 minutes until fragrant and brightly-coloured (i.e. not so frozen). Add a quarter cup of water and replace wok lid. Steam on high heat for 3 minutes.
2. Open the wok lid and splash on the Shaoxing wine. Stir again at high heat for 30 seconds to a minute to make sure the wine is cooked. Switch off and remove from heat immediately to stop overcooking.
3. Serve hot on its own or with cauliflower rice for a low carb meal or with brown rice, wholewheat pasta or noodles for healthy carb alternatives.

RED BEAN SOUP (DESSERT)

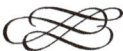

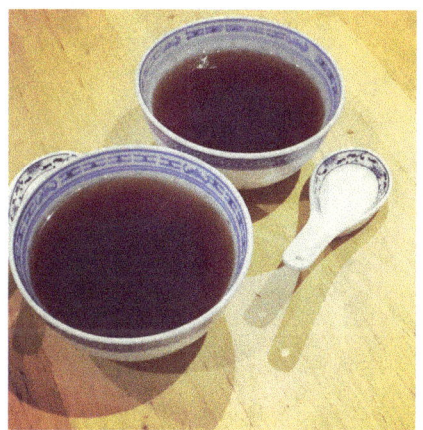

A word of caution. This is not suitable for the uninitiated white person (NSFUWP) as it's a soup served hot or chilled and it's a dessert, high in protein because of the aduki beans. I tend to make this on a very hot day for my children as I remember eating it at home after school as a thirst quencher.

It is a very traditional dessert with a popular flavour that I have grown up with. In Asia, you get red bean buns and red bean ice cream. You will need the screwpine leaves (pandan leaves) or leaves of the *Pandanus asiaticus* (it's been called the vanilla of Asia) and a bag of dried aduki beans. You can get both of these common ingredients at the Asian supermarket easily.

Serves 4-6

- 3 pandan leaves
- 1 cup of dried aduki beans (red beans)
- 3 tbsp rock sugar or caster sugar to taste if you can't get rock sugar (adjust the amount to your preference)

1. Put all of the above in the slow cooker and fill it to half full. Set it for 4 hours.
2. You can enjoy it as it is or with a splash of coconut milk mixed in.

HOW TO MAKE PERFECT RICE

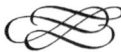

If you want to make perfect rice like you get in takeaways and restaurant meals, you need to use a rice cooker. If you cook rice in a saucepan or a pot you will end up with a) soggy rice that is a soup you have to drain away, b) soggy rice that has clumped together and become mash, c) cracked and crackly dry rice with a burnt bottom or d) a pot you have to watch all the time in order to prevent a), b) and c) from happening.

All of these problems are preventable with an automatic electric rice cooker which also frees you up to do something else.

Serves 2-4

- 2 cups of uncooked rice. **HOT TIP:** use one cup Thai fragrant white rice and one cup brown basmati rice, red rice, black rice etc for variety and nutrition
- 1 cup water

1. Put two cups of uncooked rice in the pan of the rice cooker. Wash this rice three times under the sink, each time draining off and saving the rice water for watering plants and for

washing hair, by pouring it into a medium jug and keeping aside.
2. Put the washed uncooked rice and the one cup of water in the pan into the rice cooker and switch on. While it's cooking you can do something else. In 10-12 minutes, wa-lah! You will have perfect rice.

TOP 3 ESSENTIAL DIY MARINADES, SAUCES & PASTES

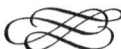

Understanding the classic Chinese flavours involves knowing some basic building blocks of making your own DIY sauces, marinades or pastes without using store-bought pre-prepared jars. You will be able to add or subtract items to these building blocks according to your likes, such as the chilli if you cannot take the heat or you love it spicy like me.

Being low fat and low sodium, home cooking is never going to be the same as a restaurant or supermarket-bought jars. It will be better — simpler and fresher, i.e. "homemade".

All these items below should be finely chopped or minced, blended or pounded into a paste-like consistency, at 1:1 ratio for any item.

You can even cheat by using a pre-made pre-made, as in the Fab Four, with its combo of shop-bought paste with fresh ingredients. Pre-mades will save you time in constructing any meal. Don't overproduce in case you never use them up. You need only small amounts each time. Keep in small jars, label their numbers (3, 4 and 5) and store inside your fridge door. Genius.

Holy Trinity

I. NGEOW

- Garlic
- Ginger
- Chilli

Fab Four

- Garlic and Ginger paste
- Sesame oil
- Shaoxing wine
- Oyster or soy sauce

Famous Five

- Chilli
- Garlic
- Ginger
- Lemongrass
- Fish sauce

LIST OF RECIPES

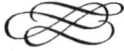

One evening, my children and I came up with the list of what we ate at home. From these and the instagram photos, the idea came about for writing this book.

1. Special fried rice
2. Egg fried rice
3. Char Siew roast pork
4. Chicken, red pepper and broccoli in oyster sauce
5. Grilled salmon, vegetables and udon noodles
6. Steamed egg and mince (Hakka egg)
7. Lemon chicken
8. Monk's vegetables (Buddha's Delight)
9. My mum's eggplant with prawn or mince
10. Shrimp bee hoon
11. Vegan bee hoon
12. My mum's Kung Pau Chi Ting (Kung Po Chicken)
13. Vegetable chow mein
14. Woh tip (pot stickers)
15. Just plain regular light and crispy tofu
16. My mum's Marmite chicken

17. Hong Kong Chinese chives omelette
18. Shrimp and Chinese cabbage tagliatelle
19. Singapore prawn mee soup noodle
20. Hakka claypot minced pork with tofu
21. Chicken chow mein
22. 3 mushroom tofu
23. Aubergine (eggplant) Thai red curry and cauliflower rice
24. My daughter's 5-ingredient chicken in 10 minutes
25. My granny's minced pork with noodles (Hakka mein)
26. Chicken macaroni soup (slow cooker)
27. Sweet and sour meatballs
28. Steamed seabass
29. Crispy roast duck with pancakes
30. Blanched pak choy
31. Beef hor fun (flat rice noodles)
32. 5-ingredient shrimp and green beans in 10 minutes
33. Red bean soup (dessert)

WANT MORE?

If you are excited by the idea of entertaining at home but don't know where to start, *Quick and Easy Party Treats: for Special Occasions* is perfect for busy beginners. Includes photos of each dish, 5 modern appetizers anyone can prepare, and a bonus original Asian-inspired cocktail. Read *Quick and Easy Party Treats: for Special Occasions*.

BEFORE YOU GO

The book you are holding in your hand is the result of my dream to be an author. I hope you enjoyed it as much as I enjoyed writing it. I am slowly building my author brand, ranking and profile. As you probably suspected, it takes weeks, months or years to write a book. It exists through dedication, passion and love. Reviews help persuade others to give my books a shot. More readers will motivate me to write, which means more books. I love connecting with and hearing from you. I personally read each review you write. It gives me a sense of fulfilment and meaning— you read my book, I read your review. It will take *less than a minute* and can be only a line to say what you liked or didn't. If you could do me just this one favour and help me, I would be ever so grateful. Please leave me a review on Amazon USA or Amazon UK. A big thank you. *Ivy*

ABOUT THE AUTHOR

I. Ngeow was born and raised in Johor Bahru, Malaysia. A graduate of the Middlesex University Writing MA programme, Ivy won the 2005 Middlesex University Literary Press Prize out of almost 1500 entrants worldwide. Her debut *Cry of the Flying Rhino* (2017) won the 2016 International Proverse Prize.

A regular suburban London mum who likes books, wine and cake, Ivy has had a passion for creative writing since she was a child, winning her first competition at 16. She started writing non-fiction lifestyle books to help families or busy and tired people, like herself, to save time and money by cooking and keeping fit at home in modern, quick and easy ways. Her interests include impromptu virtuoso piano performances, health and fitness, beauty and sewing. You can find her here:

writengeow (www.writengeow.com)
Twitter (twitter.com/ivyngeow)
Facebook (facebook.com/ivyngeowwriter)
Instagram (www.instagram.com/ivyngeow)
Email: ivy_ngeow AT yahoo DOT com

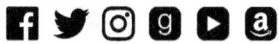

ALSO BY I. NGEOW

COOKBOOKS

Quick and Easy Party Treats: for special occasions

FITNESS

Fitness and Meal Plan Journal: 12-week daily workout and food planner notebook

Amazing at 50: 10-day Flat Tummy Challenge

Awesome at 50: Body Reboot in 6 weeks

DESIGN

Midcentury Modern: 15 Interior Design Ideas

ACKNOWLEDGMENTS

I would like to thank my publisher Leopard Print, for being "paws on" in the process, taking a chance and sinking their sharp teeth into what I think is a handy little book for new and experienced cooks. Helen Oon for taking the time to write the foreword.

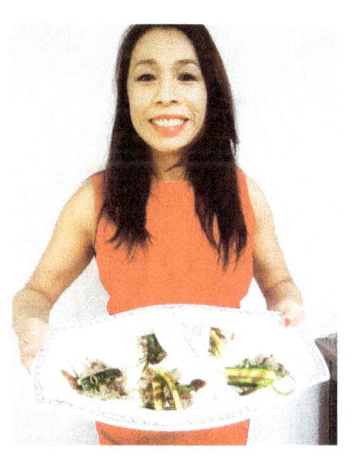

My parents both for their interest in keeping active both physically and mentally, my mother for her lifelong interest in cooking and sportsmanship in her youth. My father whose practice in and devotion to the medical profession inspired my own passion for health and fitness. My late Hakka and Hokkien grandmothers for the humble, simple and frugal meals that I grew up with, which taught me time- and money-saving tips from their own life of hardship. My family for liking what I do, how I do things and for being my original tasters (my children especially, whose favourite meals are in this book). My friends who have been invited for dinner, and who have invited me back numerous times.

You are all my teachers. You have all made every meal special. To all of you, my immense thanks.

PHOTO CREDITS

All photos belong to Ivy Ngeow except for the following which are credited as follows:

Egg fried rice by Helen Yang, Prawn Mee by su-lin, Prawn Mee with blue cloth by su-lin, Shrimp and cabbage by yummysmellsca , Steamed seabass by ehpien

www.ingramcontent.com/pod-product-compliance
Lightning Source LLC
Chambersburg PA
CBHW071740080526
44588CB00013B/2103